The fantastic Interleukins

Role in health and disease

Author – Editor: Juan Carlos Aldave

Jr. Domingo Cueto 371, Dpto. 301, Lince

Lima – Perú

Phone: (+51) 948-323-720

jucapul_84@hotmail.com

COPYRIGHT. Do not reproduce totally or partially this book without permission.

First Edition: February 2017

ISBN: 978-1546936640

February 2017

Since we are born, many dangerous microbes and malignant cells threaten our life. Therefore, we need to have powerful cells and molecules capable of defending us. We will call *immune system* to our body defenses, and *immunocytes* to the immune cells that protect us.

Our immunocytes are very strong to attack threatening organisms and cells. However, they tolerate certain molecules such as self proteins, good microbes, food and harmless substances.

Immunocytes communicate between them and with other cells through proteins called *interleukins*. In this book we will learn in a very simple and didactic way about our 38 interleukins and their role in health and disease.

Index

Chapter 1	Yola and Tola, the interleukins 1α and 1β	5
	Juan Carlos Aldave, MD	
Chapter 2	Elva, the interleukin 2	7
	Juan Carlos Aldave, MD	
Chapter 3	Mili, the interleukin 3	9
	Juan Carlos Aldave, MD; Hilda Deza, MD; Janett Díaz, MD	
Chapter 4	Sabri, the interleukin 4	11
	Juan Carlos Aldave, MD	
Chapter 5	Ale, the interleukin 5	13
	Juan C Aldave, MD; Héctor Núñez, MD; Nadia Herrera, MD	
Chapter 6	Lucy, the interleukin 6	15
	Juan Carlos Aldave, MD; Aldo Munayco, MD	
Chapter 7	Betsy, the interleukin 7	17
	Juan Carlos Aldave, MD; Joel Calero, MD	
Chapter 8	Silvia, the interleukin 8	19
	Juan Carlos Aldave, MD; Ana Alvites, MD	
Chapter 9	Elen, the interleukin 9	21
	Juan Carlos Aldave, MD	
Chapter 10	Ruth, the interleukin 10	23
	Iris Hidalgo, MD; Juan Carlos Aldave, MD	
Chapter 11	Julia, the interleukin 11	25
	Juan Carlos Aldave, MD	
Chapter 12	Bolli, the interleukin 12	27
	Juan Carlos Aldave, MD	

Chapter 13	Marce, the interleukin 13	**29**
	Juan Carlos Aldave, MD; Jesús Andrade, MD	
Chapter 14	Iris, the interleukin 14	**31**
	Juan Carlos Aldave, MD	
Chapter 15	Vicki, the interleukin 15	**33**
	Juan Carlos Aldave, MD	
Chapter 16	Jess, the interleukin 16	**35**
	Juan Carlos Aldave, MD	
Chapter 17	Anne, the interleukin 17A, and their sisters	**37**
	Juan Carlos Aldave, MD	
Chapter 18	Pia, the interleukin 18	**39**
	Juan Carlos Aldave, MD	
Chapter 19	Vane, the interleukin 19	**41**
	Juan Carlos Aldave, MD	
Chapter 20	Kate, the interleukin 20	**43**
	Juan Carlos Aldave, MD	
Chapter 21	Lisa, the interleukin 21	**45**
	Juan Carlos Aldave, MD	
Chapter 22	Sami, the interleukin 22	**47**
	Juan Carlos Aldave, MD	
Chapter 23	Mari, the interleukin 23	**49**
	Juan Carlos Aldave, MD	
Chapter 24	Lila, the interleukin 24	**51**
	Juan Carlos Aldave, MD	
Chapter 25	Flor, the interleukin 25	**53**
	Juan Carlos Aldave, MD	

Chapter 26	Shen, the interleukin 26	**55**
	Juan Carlos Aldave, MD	
Chapter 27	Luna, the interleukin 27	**57**
	Juan Carlos Aldave, MD	
Chapter 28	Lili y Lali, the interleukins 28A and 28B	**59**
	Juan Carlos Aldave, MD	
Chapter 29	Areli, the interleukin 29	**61**
	Juan Carlos Aldave, MD	
Chapter 30	Fanny, the interleukin 30	**63**
	Juan Carlos Aldave, MD	
Chapter 31	Rachel, the interleukin 31	**65**
	Juan Carlos Aldave, MD	
Chapter 32	Gabi, the interleukin 32	**67**
	Juan Carlos Aldave, MD	
Chapter 33	Techi, the interleukin 33	**69**
	Juan Carlos Aldave, MD	
Chapter 34	Gina, the interleukin 34	**71**
	Juan Carlos Aldave, MD	
Chapter 35	Carla, the interleukin 35	**73**
	Juan Carlos Aldave, MD	
Chapter 36	Adela, the interleukin 36	**75**
	Juan Carlos Aldave, MD	
Chapter 37	Ethel, the interleukin 37	**77**
	Juan Carlos Aldave, MD	
Chapter 38	Gladys, the interleukin 38	**79**
	Juan Carlos Aldave, MD	

Yola and Tola, IL-1α and IL-1β

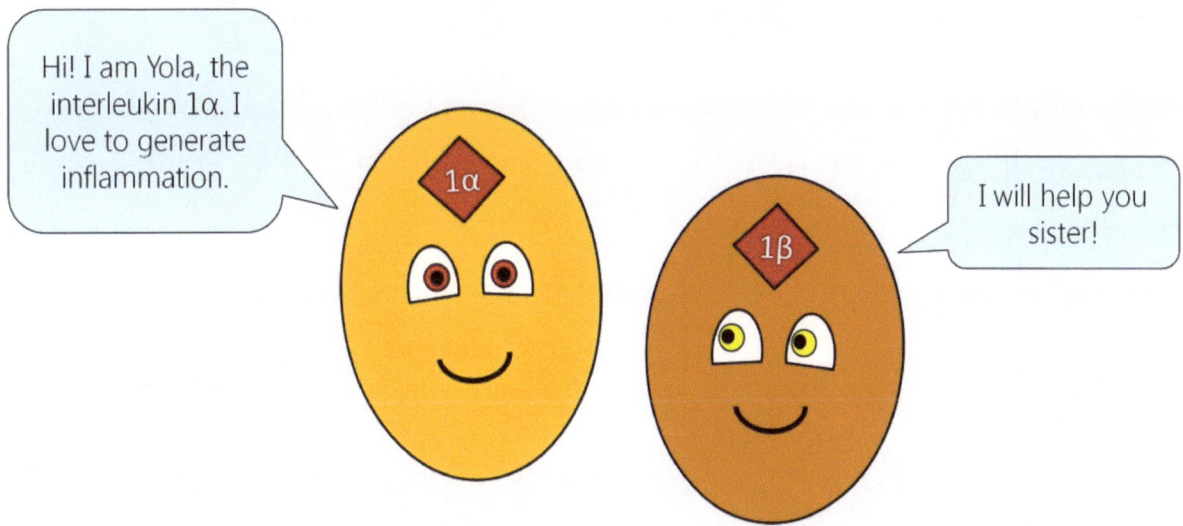

The family of interleukin 1 is composed of eleven cytokines: seven are inflammatory (IL-1α, IL-1β, IL-18, IL-33, IL-36α, IL-36β, IL-36γ) and the other 4 are antiinflammatory (IL-1Ra, IL-36Ra, IL-37, IL-38).

IL-1α and IL-1β have potent inflammatory activity. Their natural antagonist is the protein IL-1Ra (interleukin 1 receptor antagonist).

Where are they produced?

Yola and Tola are produced primarily by activated macrophages. Their actions are proinflammatory and pyrogenic. IL-1β also favors the differentiation of TH17 lymphocytes.

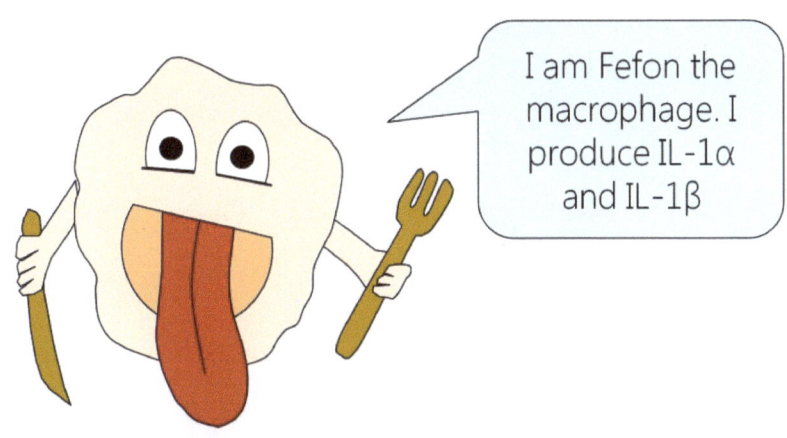

Are there people who cannot produce IL-1α or IL-1β?

So far there are no reports of subjects with pathogenic mutations in the genes encoding IL-1α and IL-1β.

However, there are patients who cannot synthesize the antagonist molecule IL-1Ra. The resulting disease is called DIRA (Deficiency of the Interleukin 1 Receptor Antagonist), characterized by multifocal osteomyelitis, periostitis and pustulosis of neonatal onset.

Are there people who produce IL-1α or IL-1β in excess?

Yes, excessive production of IL-1α and IL-1β occurs in:

- Many autoimmune diseases such as rheumatoid arthritis, psoriasis and inflammatory bowel disease.
- Several autoinflammatory disorders (genetic defects that generate disproportionate activation of innate immunity), such as Familiar Mediterranean fever and Muckle-Wells syndrome.

In patients with these diseases both cytokines become therapeutic targets. For example:

- The drug Anakinra is a synthetic antagonist of IL-1.
- The monoclonal antibody Canakinumab traps IL-1β.

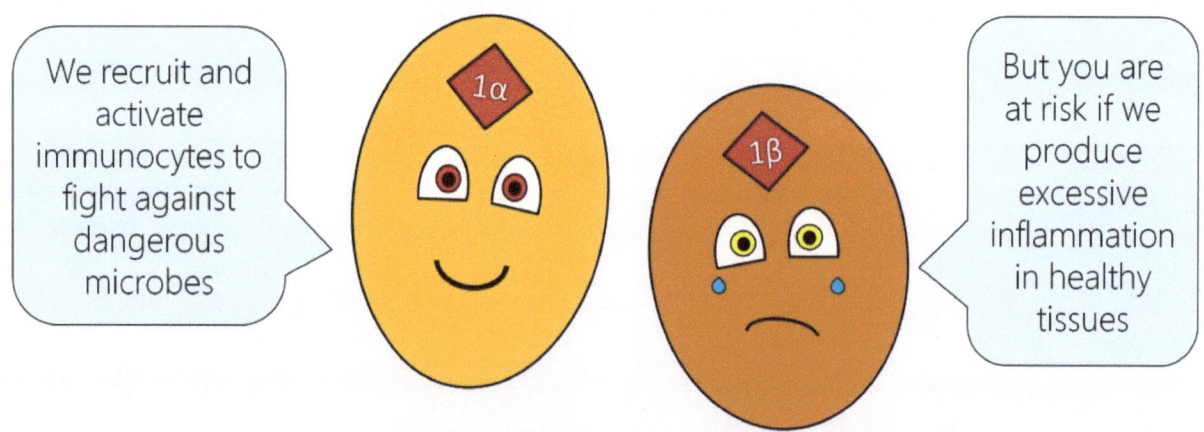

Elva, the interleukin 2

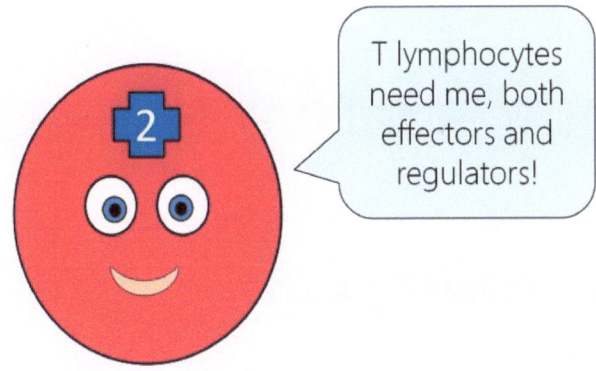

Elva is an essential protein for T lymphocytes. Its receptor (IL-2R) is formed by 3 chains: IL-2Rα (CD25), IL-2Rβ and IL-2Rγ (CD132, γc or gamma common chain). γc is also part of the receptors of interleukins 4, 7, 9, 15 and 21.

Where is Elva produced?

IL-2, fabricated initially by dendritic cells, stimulates the activation of T lymphocytes. Activated T cells synthesize more IL-2 and IL-2R, amplifying their proliferation in an autocrine fashion.

On the other hand, IL-2 at low doses is essential for the development of regulatory T lymphocytes. Elva also participates in the activation of innate lymphoid cells, B lymphocytes and NK cells.

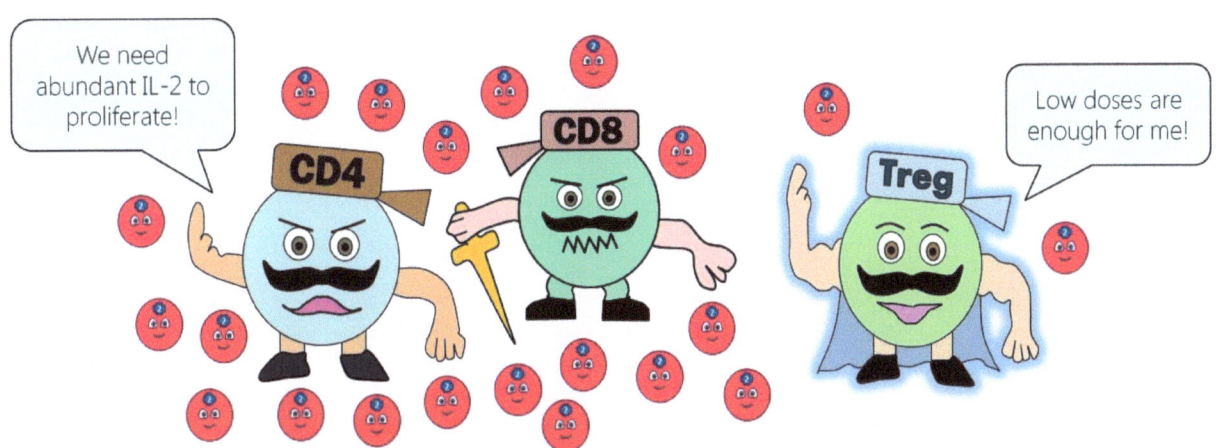

Are there people who cannot produce IL-2 or its receptor?

γc deficiency causes an absence of T lymphocytes (lack of response to IL-2 and IL-7) and NK cells (lack of response to IL-15), giving rise to severe combined immunodeficiency. Affected patients are susceptible to infections by all kinds of microbes.

The absence of IL-2Rα prevents the activation of effector and regulatory T cells, favoring infectious and autoimmune processes.

High-dose recombinant IL-2 can potentiate effector T lymphocytes in subjects with immunodeficiencies, cancer, or chronic infections. At low doses, IL-2 could attenuate autoimmunity by promoting differentiation of regulatory T lymphocytes.

Are there people who fabricate IL-2 in excess?

Excessive IL-2 activity may favor the development of autoimmune diseases such as multiple sclerosis.

IL-2 activates T lymphocytes in patients receiving an allogeneic transplant, favoring the rejection of foreign tissue. In this context, anti-IL2Rα monoclonal antibodies (e.g. daclizumab, basiliximab) reduce rejection risk.

Denileukin diftitox (recombinant IL-2 joined to Diphtheria toxin) is a compound that can be useful in T cell neoplasms.

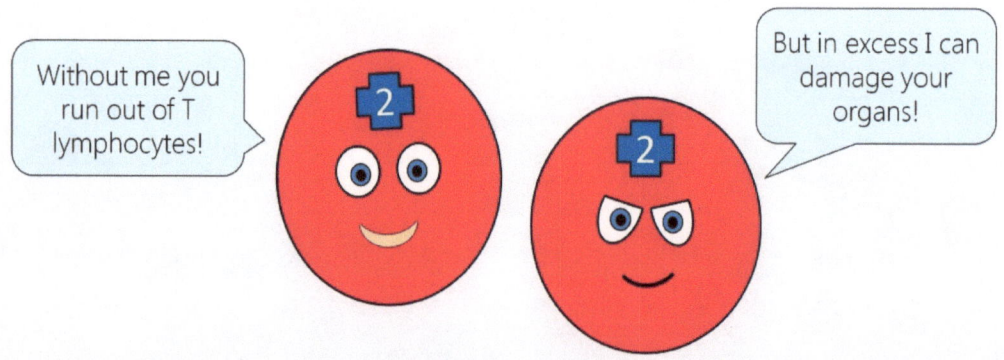

Mili, the interleukin 3

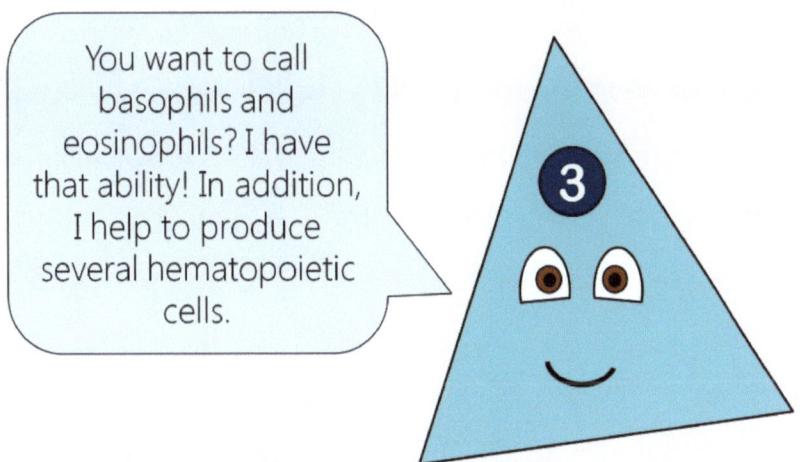

IL-3 is a hematopoietic growth factor that stimulates the production of several blood cell lineages. It also has the ability to activate basophils and eosinophils.

Where is Mili produced?

Mili is produced by T lymphocytes, especially TH2 cells, macrophages, NK cells, certain stromal cells, mast cells and eosinophils.

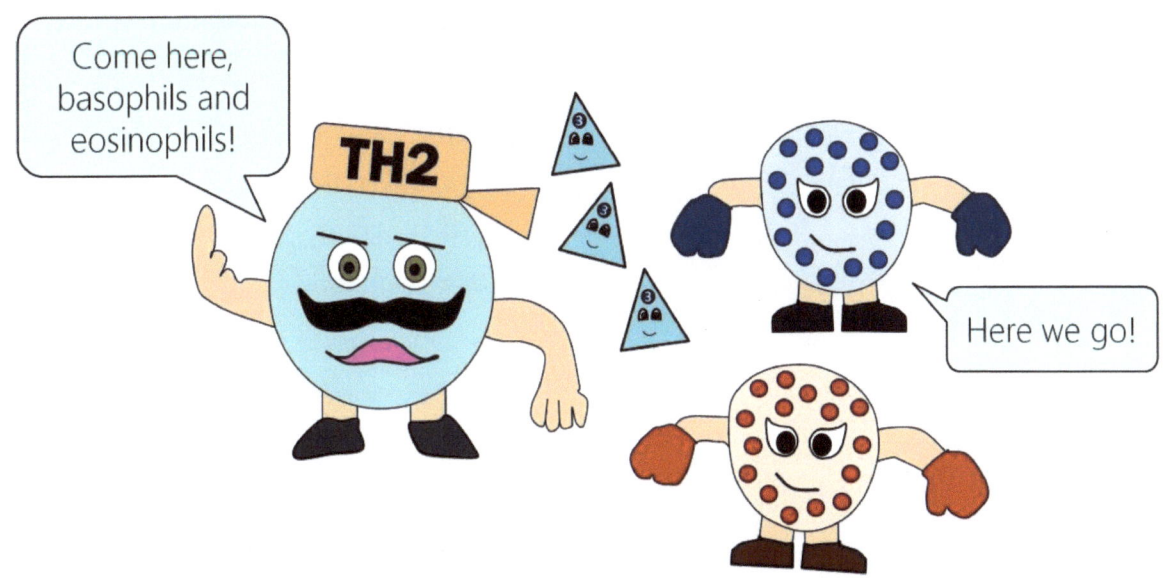

Are there people who cannot produce IL-3?

So far, human beings with clinically relevant mutations in the IL-3 gene have not been described

However, genetically modified mice deficient in IL-3 could have a reduction in the number of mast cells and basophils, as well as a decreased immune response to helminth parasites (e.g. *Strongyloides venezuelensis*).

In patients with cancer-related myelosuppression, the application of IL-3 as a stimulant of hematopoiesis has been investigated.

Are there people who fabricate IL-3 in excess?

Yes. In individuals with IgE-mediated allergic diseases (e.g. allergic rhinitis, bronchial asthma), TH2 lymphocytes recruit inflammatory basophils and eosinophils through the production of IL-3 and other cytokines.

Currently, IL-3 is not considered a therapeutic target for allergic diseases.

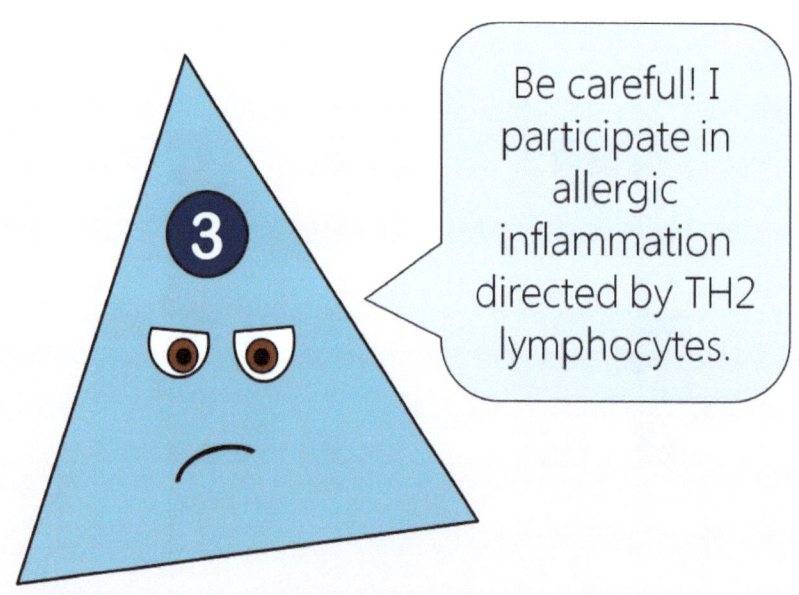

Sabri, the interleukin 4

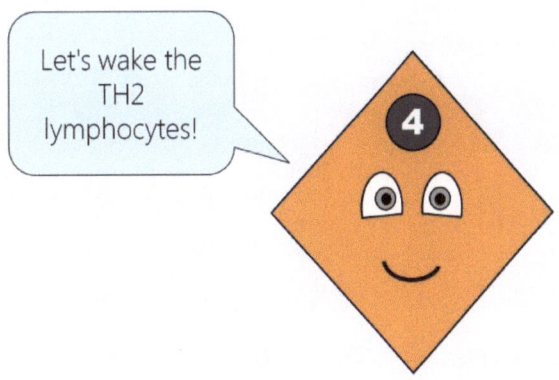

Sabri is a cytokine that induces TH2 immunity through 2 receptors: a) type 1 receptor, formed by IL-4Rα chain and the common gamma chain; b) type 2 receptor, formed by IL-4Rα chain and IL-13Rα chain (IL-13 also signals through this type 2 receptor).

Where is Sabri produced?

The main sources of IL-4 are TH2 lymphocytes, type 2 innate lymphoid cells (ILC2), basophils, mast cells and eosinophils. Sabri strengthens our TH2 army against helminths and other extracellular parasites by inducing the development of TH2 lymphocytes and the secretion of IgE from B lymphocytes.

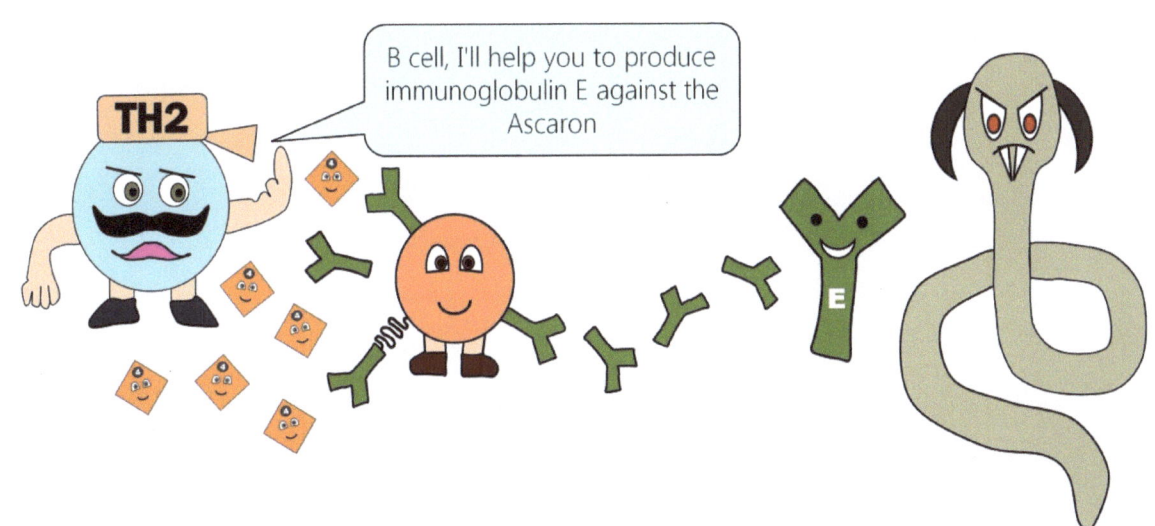

Are there people who cannot produce IL-4?

No human immunodeficiencies have been described because of the absence of IL-4.

Are there people who fabricate IL-4 in excess?

Yes, excessive production of IL-4 against molecules that should be tolerated favors the development of TH2 allergic diseases, such as allergic bronchial asthma, allergic rhinitis and atopic dermatitis.

In patients with these diseases, IL-4 and its receptor are therapeutic targets for novel drugs. For example:

- The drug Pitrakinra is a mutated recombinant version of IL-4 that binds to the IL-4Rα subunit, thereby blocking the action of interleukins 4 and 13.
- Pascolizumab is a humanized anti-IL-4 monoclonal antibody investigated as an asthma therapy.
- The monoclonal antibody Dupilumab is directed against the IL-4Rα subunit of the IL-4 receptor. It blocks the activity of IL-4 and IL-13, becoming one of the most promising drugs for the treatment of TH2 allergies.

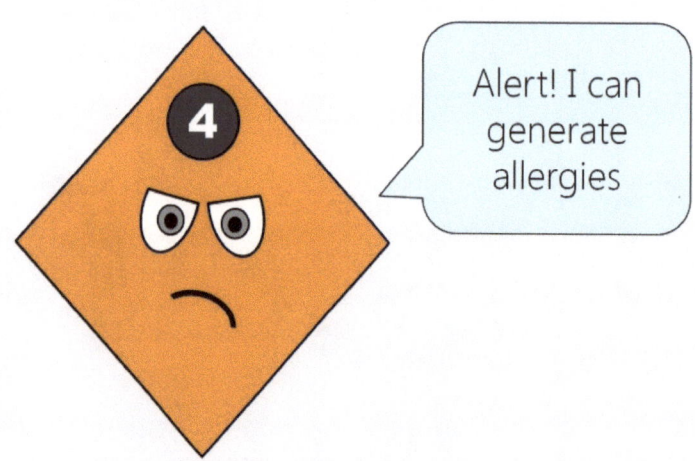

Ale, the interleukin 5

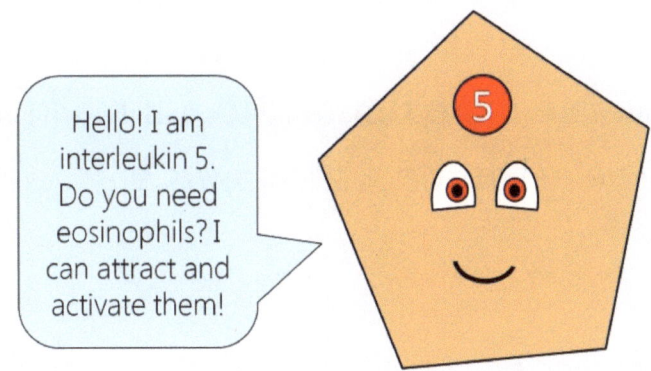

IL-5 belongs to the group of TH2 cytokines. Its receptor is a heterodimer formed by an alpha chain (IL-5Rα) and a beta chain (βc). βc is also part of the IL-3 and GM-CSF receptor.

IL-5 is produced during the TH2 immune response against worms such as the Ascaron (*Ascaris lumbricoides*). This cytokine promotes the proliferation, activation, survival and adhesion of eosinophils. It also participates in tissue remodeling and repair.

Where is Ale produced?

Ale is produced mainly by CD4 TH2 lymphocytes, type 2 innate lymphoid cells (ILC2), activated eosinophils and mast cells.

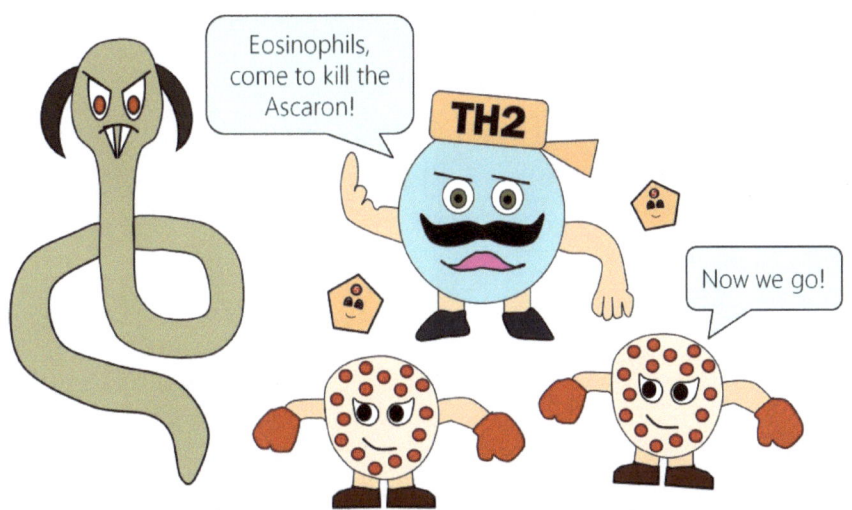

Are there people who cannot produce IL-5?

Human immunodeficiencies due to the absence of IL-5 have not been described yet.

IL-5-deficient mice are more resistant to asthma induction and less able to expel the helminth *Nippostrongylus brasiliensis*.

Are there people who fabricate IL-5 in excess?

Yes, excessive producción of IL-5 occurs in patients with:

- Eosinophilic asthma, where eosinophils contribute to airway inflammation as well as tissue destruction and remodeling.

- Other eosinophilic diseases, such as eosinophilic esophagitis and gastroenteritis, hypereosinophilic syndromes, etc.).

In these inflammatory diseases, IL-5 becomes a therapeutic target. For example:

- Anti-IL-5 monoclonal antibodies (Mepolizumab and Reslizumab) are potentially beneficial for patients with eosinophilic diseases.
- Benralizumab, a monoclonal antibody directed against IL-5Rα, has the same potential.

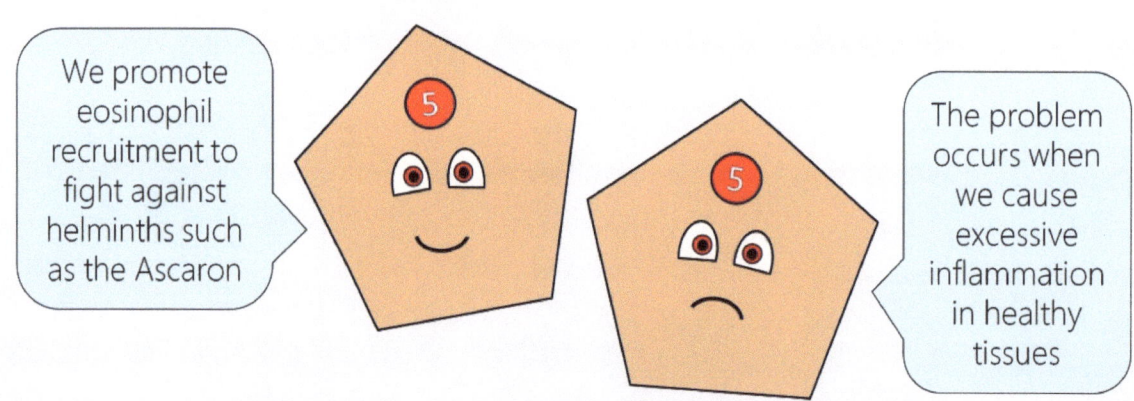

Lucy, the interleukin 6

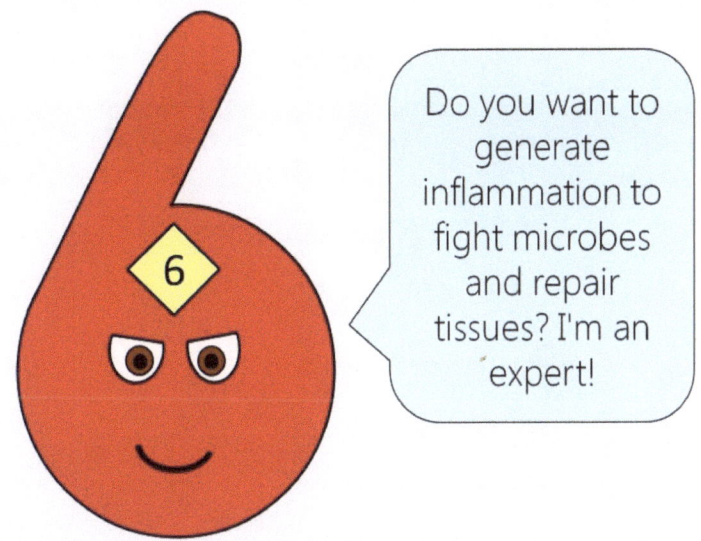

Lucy belongs to the family of cytokines 'IL-6-type', which includes leukemia inhibitory factor, ciliary neurotrophic factor and oncostatin M. Its receptor consists of an IL-6 binding chain (IL-6Rα) and the signaling component gp130.

Lucy is a multifunctional cytokine with essentially inflammatory actions:

- Stimulates hepatic production of acute-phase reactants.

- Induces hematopoiesis.

- Recruits and activates phagocytes.

- Induces the differentiation and activation of T and B cells.

- Promotes the differentiation of T CD4 lymphocytes into TH17 lymphocytes, the commanders of our immune army against extracellular fungi and bacteria such as *Candida albicans* and *Staphylococcus aureus*.

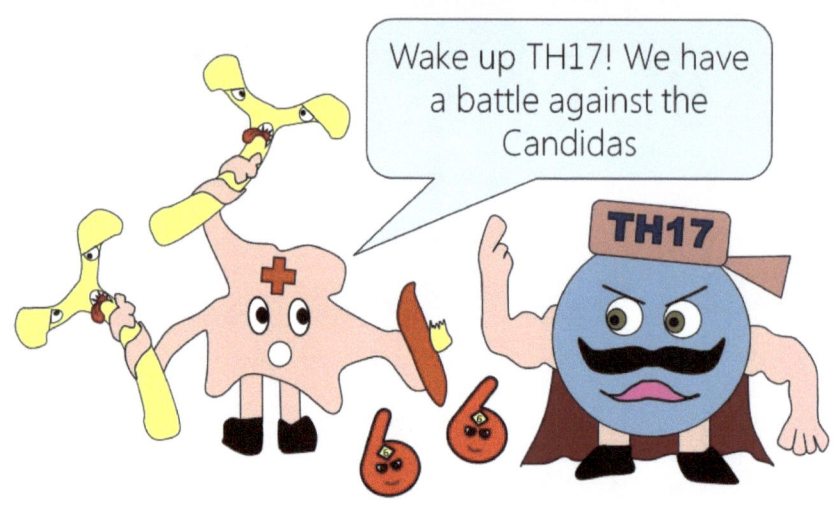

Where is Lucy produced?

Lucy is produced by macrophages, endothelial cells and fibroblasts.

Are there people who cannot produce IL-6?

Some individuals produce neutralizing antibodies against IL-6, becoming susceptible to infections by *Staphylococcus aureus*.

Are there people who fabricate IL-6 in excess?

Yes, excess production of IL-6 occurs in patients with certain autoimmune or autoinflammatory diseases such as rheumatoid arthritis and systemic lupus erythematosus.

Patients affected by these diseases may improve with Tocilizumab, a monoclonal antibody against the IL-6 receptor.

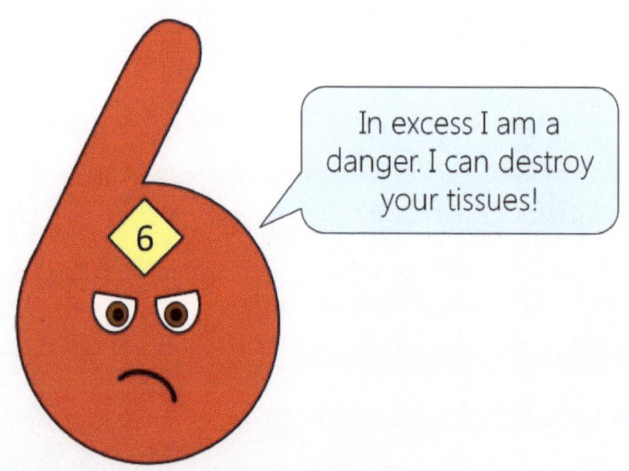

Betsy, the interleukin 7

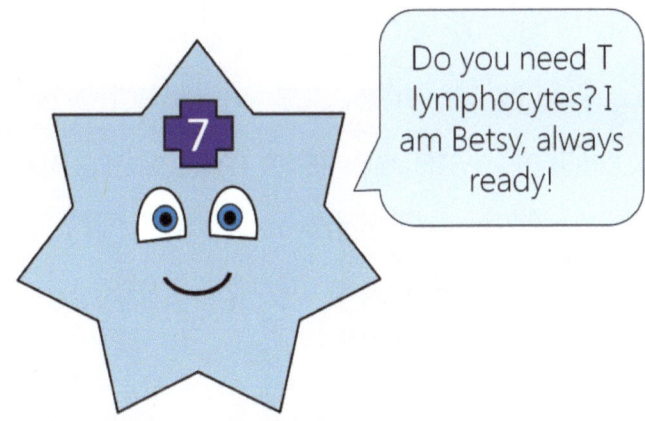

The main function of IL-7 in humans is to activate T lymphocytes. Betsy acts through its receptor composed of an alpha chain (IL-7Rα or CD127) and the common gamma chain (γc or CD132).

Where is Betsy produced?

IL-7 is synthesized by dendritic cells, B lymphocytes, monocytes/macrophages and epithelial cells including keratinocytes. Betsy induces the development, proliferation and survival of T lymphocytes. It also favors the development and maintenance of innate lymphoid cells (ILCs).

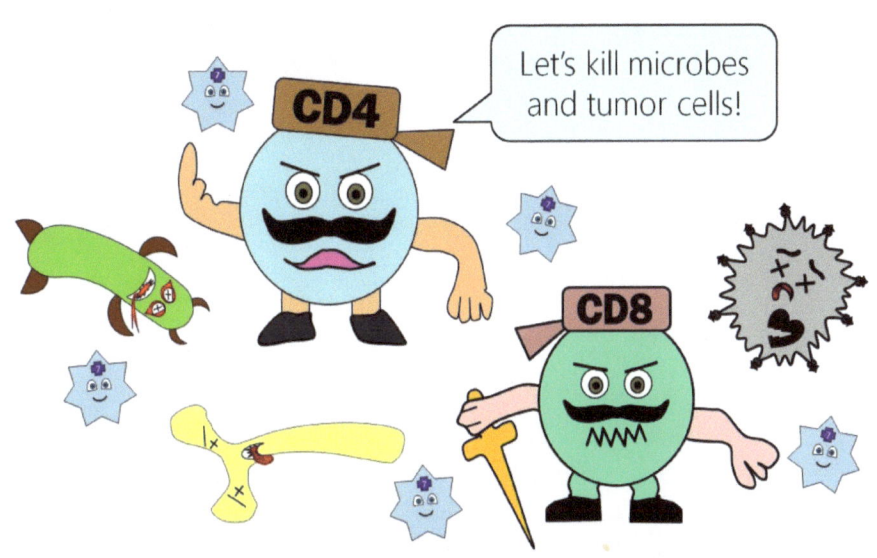

Are there people who cannot produce IL-7?

Patients with genetic defects in IL-7Rα cannot fabricate T lymphocytes, resulting in severe combined immunodeficiency (SCID) with susceptibility to all types of infections. The problem is even greater in children with genetic mutations in γc, who cannot produce NK cells neither. Children with SCID need urgently a hematopoietic stem cell transplant or gene therapy to survive.

Human recombinant IL-7 can empower T lymphocytes in patients with cancer, AIDS, chronic viral infections, or post-transplant immunodeficiency.

Are there people who fabricate IL-7 in excess?

Excessive activation of T lymphocytes induced by IL-7 can occur in several autoimmune and inflammatory diseases such as multiple sclerosis, type 1 diabetes, rheumatoid arthritis, sarcoidosis or graft-versus-host disease.

Could IL-7 be a therapeutic target in these diseases? Probably yes. The problem would be the immunodeficiency generated by blocking the action of IL-7.

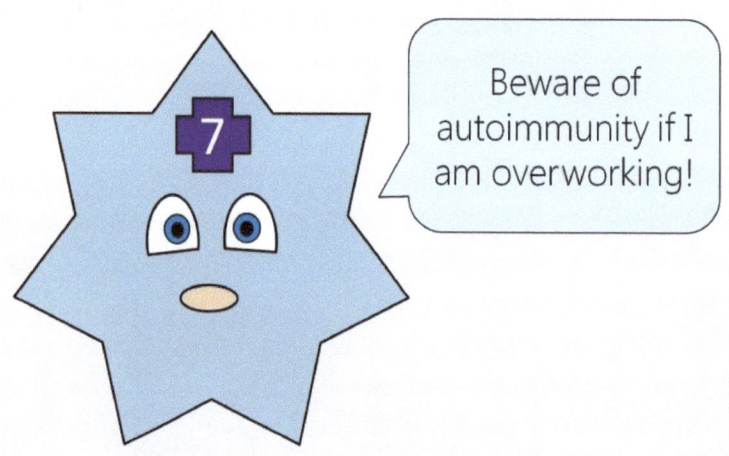

Silvia, the interleukin 8

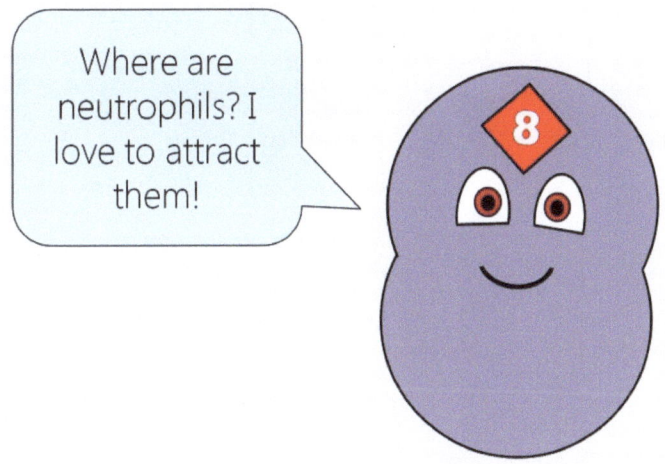

Silvia belongs to the CXC chemokine family. It acts through its receptors CXCR1 (IL-8RA) and CXCR2 (IL-8RB).

Where is Silvia produced?

Several cells make IL-8 (macrophages, lymphocytes, neutrophils, endothelial and epithelial cells), especially after stimulation with IL-1α, IL-1β, IL-17 or TNF-α. Its main function is to recruit neutrophils to sites of infection or damage. It can also attract T and NK lymphocytes, basophils and eosinophils. It promotes angiogenesis.

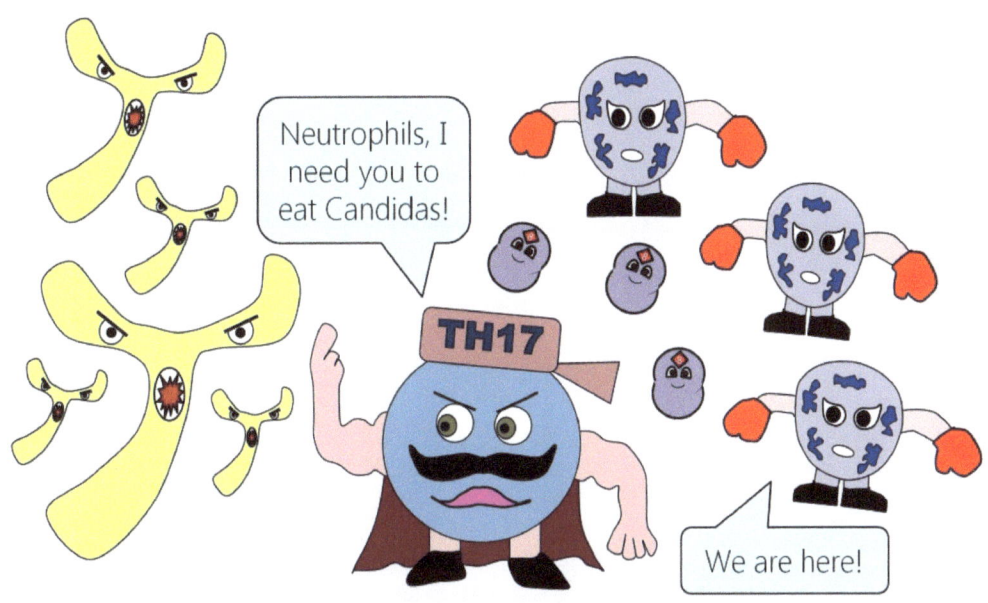

Are there people who cannot produce IL-8?

Genetic defects affecting TH17 immunity (e.g. STAT1 gain-of-function, CARD9 deficiency) reduce the ability to synthesize IL-8 and recruit neutrophils, leading to increased susceptibility to infections by extracellular fungi and bacteria.

Are there people who fabricate IL-8 in excess?

Yes. Excessive production of IL-8 generates damage. This occurs in chronic inflammatory diseases such as rheumatoid arthritis, psoriasis, chronic obstructive pulmonary disease (COPD), neutrophilic asthma and various neoplasms.

Clinical trials with anti-IL-8 monoclonal antibodies (HuMax-IL-8, ABX-IL-8) have been performed in inflammatory diseases such as palmoplantar pustulosis, COPD and cancer. Theoretically, any disease where tissue damage is caused by neutrophils could improve antagonizing the action of IL-8.

Polymorphisms in the IL-8 gene may increase the risk of atrophic gastritis and gastric cancer caused by a local excess of IL-8 and neutrophilic infiltration.

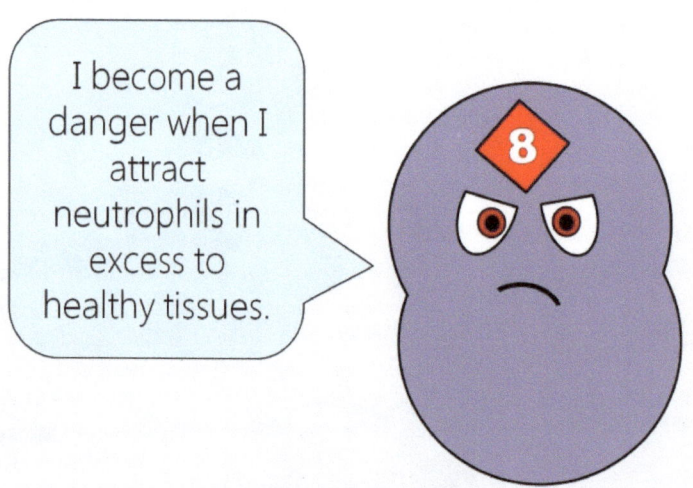

Elen, the interleukin 9

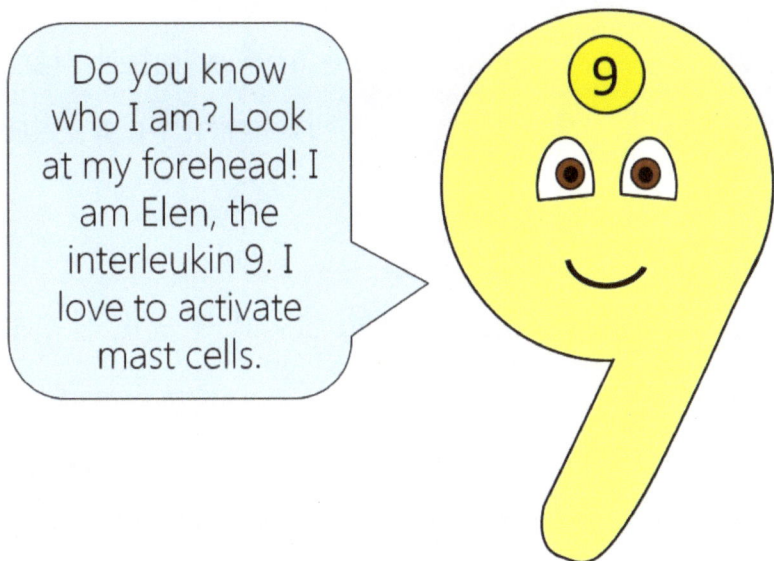

IL-9 is a proinflammatory cytokine whose receptor is formed by an IL-9Rα chain and the common gamma chain (γc).

Where is Elen produced?

Elen is mainly synthesized by TH2 and TH9 lymphocytes, type 2 innate lymphoid cells (ILC2), mast cells and eosinophils.

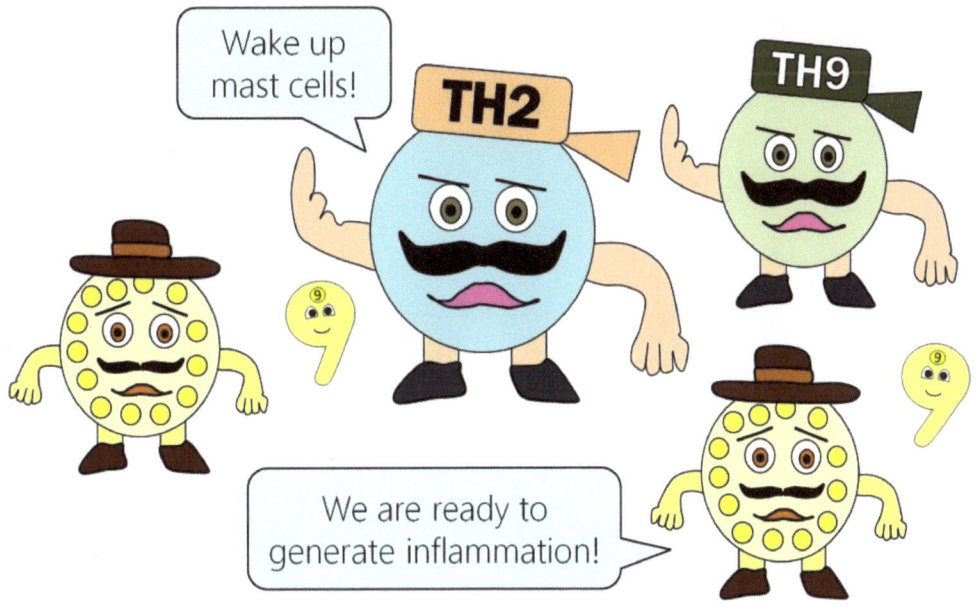

The main action of IL-9 is to stimulate the production and activation of mast cells. In addition, it increases secretion of mucus by epithelial cells and favors IgE synthesis.

Physiologically, these actions promote immediate inflammation and activation of our TH2 army to combat helminth parasites.

Are there people who cannot produce IL-9?

Patients with clinically significant defects in the IL-9 gene have not been described.

Are there people who fabricate IL-9 in excess?

Unfortunately yes. In patients with IgE-mediated allergic diseases (eg, allergic rhinitis, bronchial asthma), TH2 and TH9 lymphocytes, as well as ILC2, activate mast cells through IL-9 and other related cytokines.

The therapeutic effect of an anti-IL-9 monoclonal antibody is being investigated in patients with bronchial asthma.

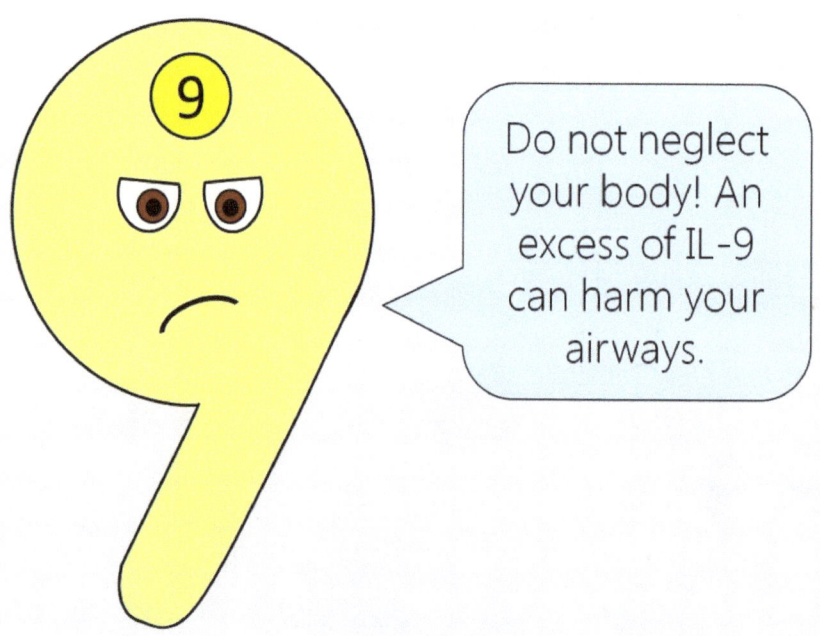

Ruth, the interleukin 10

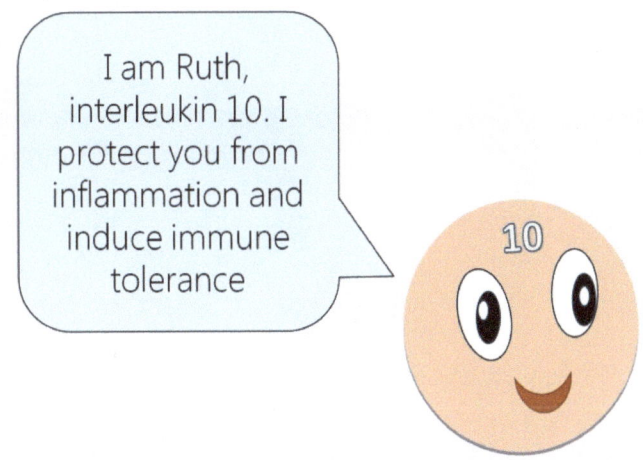

IL-10, acting on its IL-10R1/IL10R2 receptor, is an anti-inflammatory and regulatory cytokine. Together with other cytokines (IL-19, IL-20, IL-22, IL-24, IL-26, IL-28, IL-29), they compose the IL-10 family.

Where is Ruth produced?

IL-10 is synthesized by monocytes, dendritic cells and lymphocytes, particularly by the regulatory cells TR1 and B10.

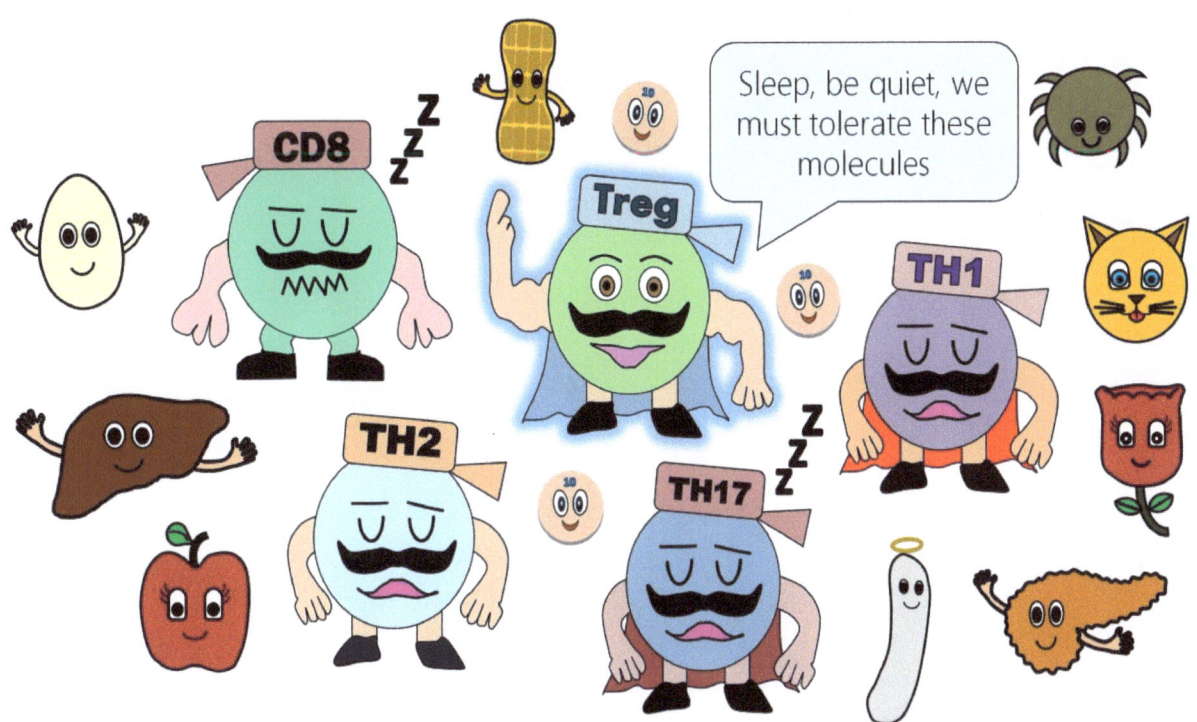

Ruth has several immunoregulatory actions. For example:

- Induces dendritic cells to a tolerogenic phenotype (↓ HLA class II molecules, ↓ proinflammatory cytokines, ↓ costimulatory molecules CD80 and CD86).

- Promotes the differentiation of T regulatory lymphocytes (TR1) and inhibits T effector lymphocytes (TH1, TH2, TH17).

- Stimulates synthesis of IgG4 by B lymphocytes.

Are there people who cannot produce IL-10?

Children with genetic defects in IL-10 or its receptor (IL-10R1/IL-10R2) suffer severe early-onset inflammation (inflammatory bowel disease with perianal fistulas, folliculitis, arthritis).

A local defect in IL-10 expression may favor the development of intestinal inflammation, autoimmunity (e.g. rheumatoid arthritis, lupus), allergies (e.g. allergic rhinitis), and neoplasms. The effect of recombinant IL-10 on these pathologies is being tested.

Are there people who fabricate IL-10 in excess?

Theoretically, local excess of IL-10 would facilitate the spread of infections and cancer. However, in real life, recombinant IL-10 appears to be useful for the treatment of malignancies.

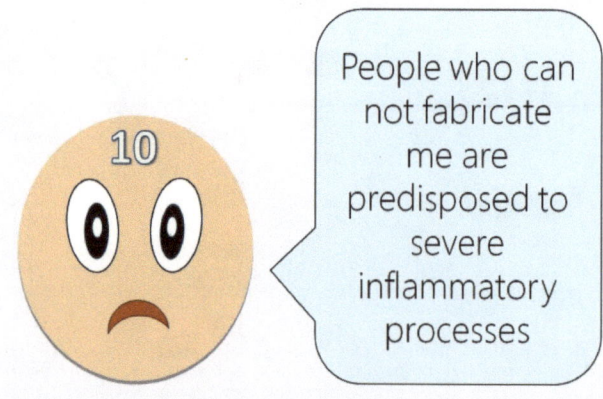

Julia, the interleukin 11

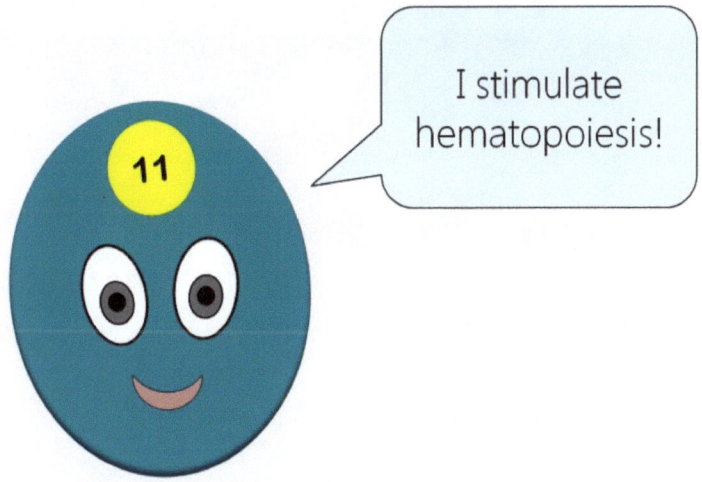

The IL-11 receptor is made up of 2 subunits: IL-11Rα and gp130. Remind that gp130 is also part of the receptors of IL-6 and other proteins (ciliary neurotrophic factor, leukemia inhibitory factor, oncostatin M and cardiotrophin-1).

Where is Julia produced?

Various cells can make IL-11, such as stromal cells of the bone marrow, fibroblasts, epithelial cells, endothelial cells, synoviocytes and osteoblasts.

The main function of Julia, in synergy with IL-3, is to stimulate hematopoiesis, fundamentally platelet production. Other functions are: protection of epithelial cells and connective tissue, induction of acute phase proteins, neuronal development, bone remodeling by stimulating osteoclasts and inhibiting osteoblasts, and activation of B lymphocytes.

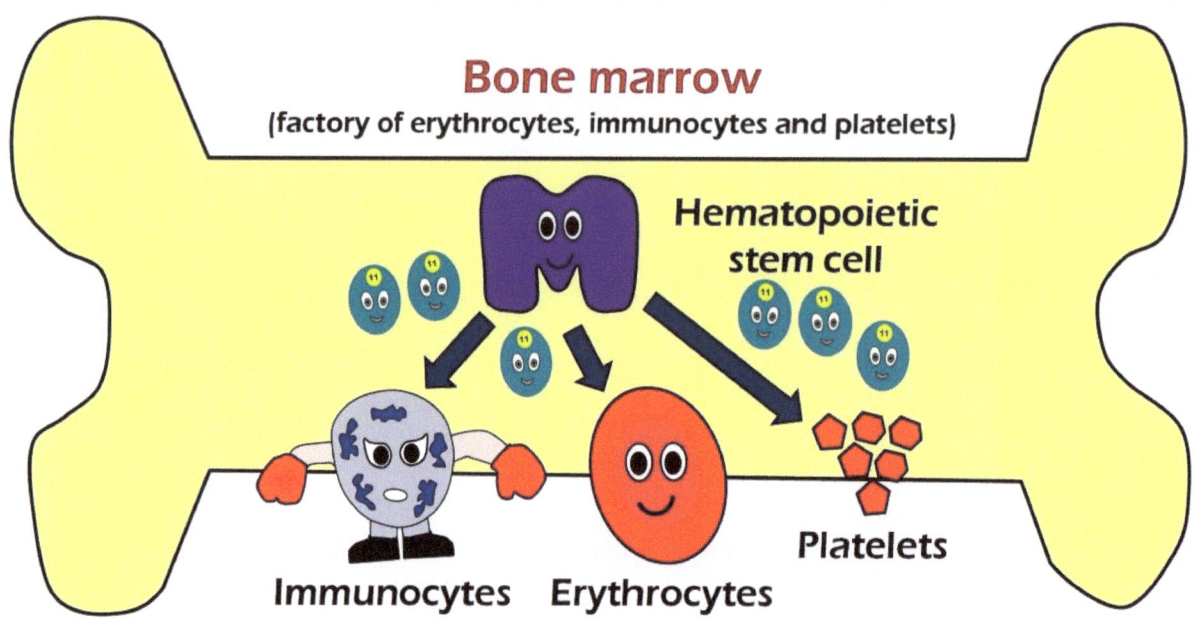

Are there people who cannot produce IL-11?

So far there are no reports of genetic diseases caused by the absence of IL-11.

Recombinant human IL-11 (Oprelvekin) stimulates platelet production and may be useful for patients with thrombocytopenia (e.g. post-chemotherapy).

Are there people who fabricate IL-11 in excess?

Certain polymorphisms in the IL-11 gene have been associated with ulcerative colitis and chronic obstructive pulmonary disease.

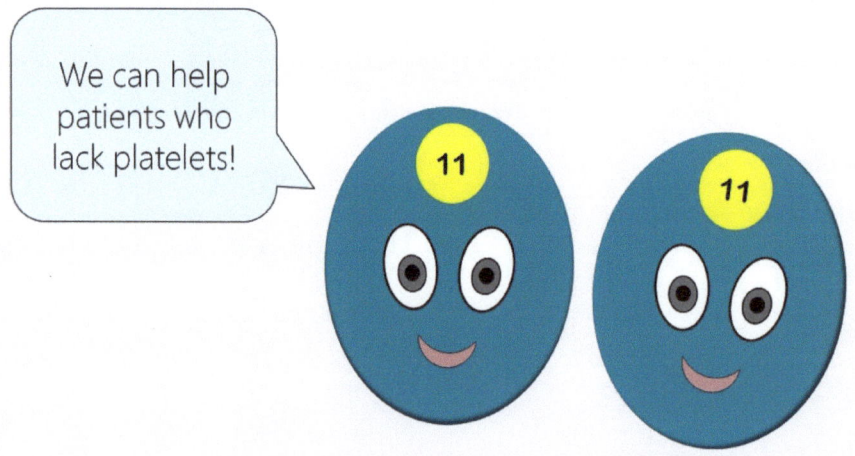

Bolli, the interleukin 12

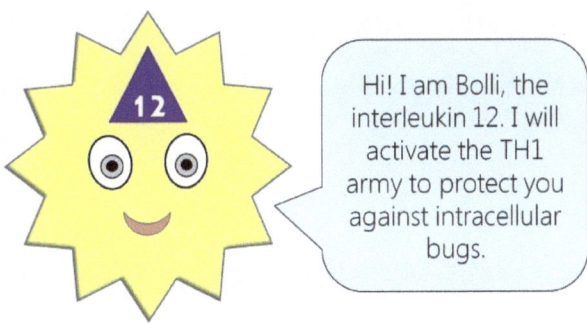

The bioactive form of IL-12 (IL-12p70) has 2 subunits: p35 and p40. The p40 subunit is also part of IL-23. The IL-12 receptor has 2 chains: IL-12Rβ1 (also makes up the IL-23 receptor) and IL-12Rβ2 (is also part of the IL-35 receptor).

Where is Bolli produced?

IL-12 is mainly synthesized by monocytes, macrophages and dendritic cells. Its major function is to activate our TH1 army against intracellular microbes (e.g. mycobacteria, *Salmonella spp*, *Histoplasma spp*, virus, etc.) and tumor cells.

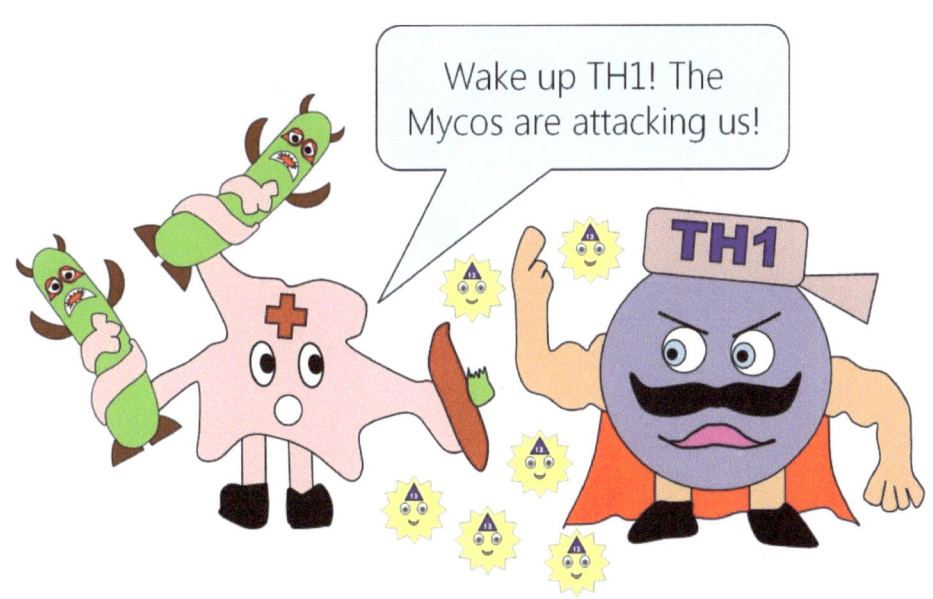

In addition to inducing the differentiation and maintenance of TH1 lymphocytes, Bolli is able to activate NK lymphocytes and type 1 innate lymphoid cells (ILC1). Activated TH1 and NK lymphocytes synthesize interferon-gamma (IFN-γ), thus enhancing the attack against intracellular microbes and malignant cells (IL-12/IFN-γ axis).

Are there people who cannot produce IL-12?

Yes. Patients with primary immunodeficiencies due to absence of IL-12p40 or IL-12Rβ1 are susceptible to infections by intracellular microbes such as mycobacteria or Salmonella (Mendelian susceptibility to mycobacterial diseases). The same problem affects subjects with deficiency of IFN-γ or its receptor.

By enhancing TH1 immunity, recombinant IL-12 is a potential treatment for subjects with immunodeficiencies or cancer.

Are there people who fabricate IL-12 in excess?

Yes. Excessive activity of our TH1 army against self molecules can lead to the onset of autoimmune diseases.

Ustekinumab is a monoclonal antibody that neutralizes the p40 subunit of IL-12 and IL-23, thereby inhibiting the activation of TH1 and TH17 immunity, respectively. Therefore, this biologic drug has therapeutic potential for autoimmune diseases such as psoriasis.

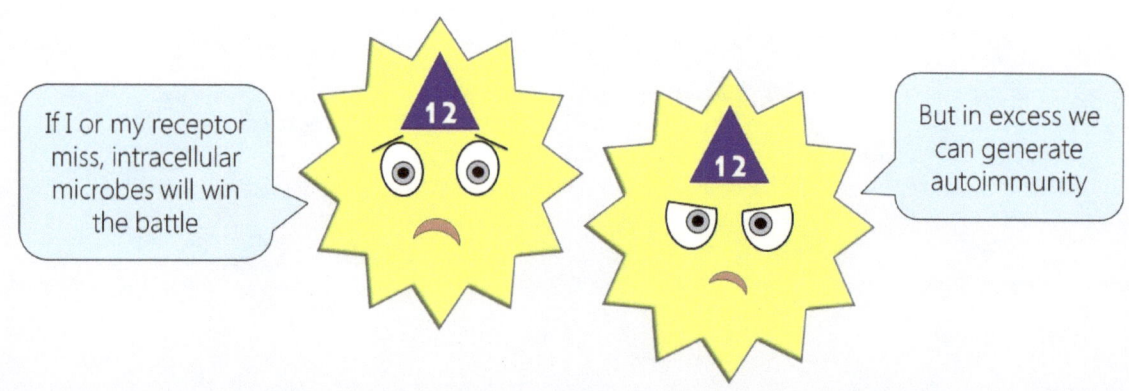

Marce, the interleukin 13

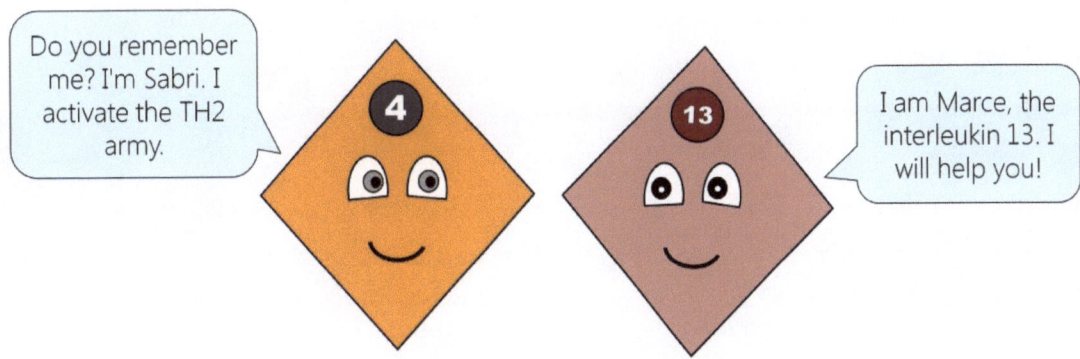

IL-13 exerts similar actions to IL-4; both cytokines induce the TH2 immune response against helminths. An important difference between them is that IL-13, unlike IL-4, does not have a receptor on T lymphocytes; therefore, IL-13 cannot directly promote the differentiation of CD4 TH2 lymphocytes.

The major receptor of IL-13 is formed by the IL-4Rα chain (it is also part of the IL-4 receptor) and the IL-13Rα1 chain.

Where is Marce produced?

Marce is synthesized by TH2 lymphocytes, type 2 innate lymphoid cells, basophils, mast cells and eosinophils. Marce amplifies the TH2 immune response through the following actions:

- Induces synthesis of IgE by B lymphocytes.
- Activates mast cells and eosinophils.
- Increases mucus production by epithelial cells.
- Stimulates smooth muscle contraction.
- Promotes tissue remodeling.

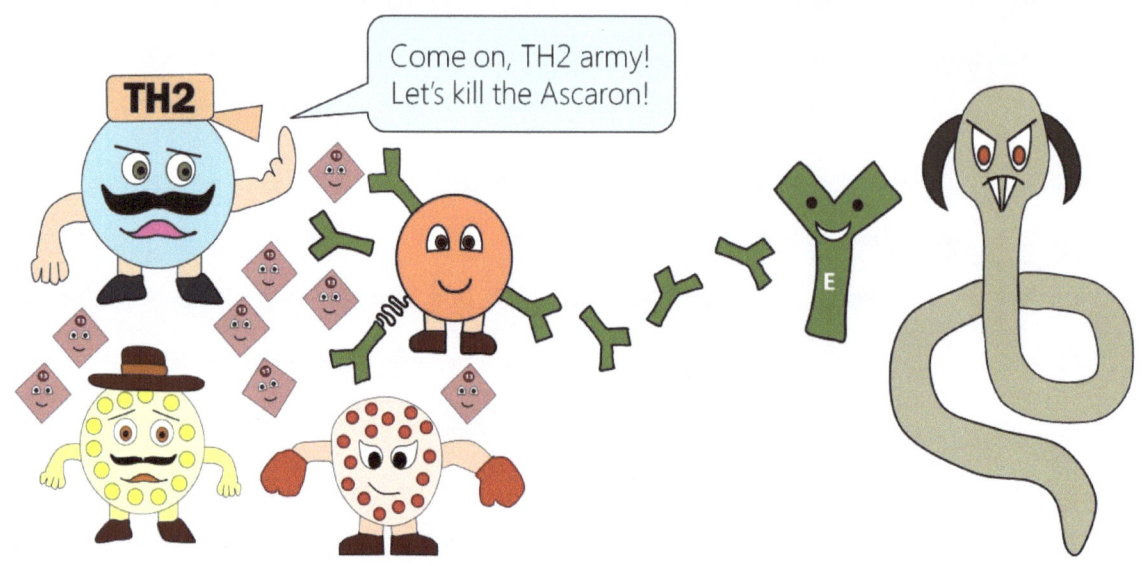

Are there people who cannot produce IL-13?

Immunodeficiencies due to lack of IL-13 have not been described.

Are there people who fabricate IL-13 in excess?

Yes, an excess of IL-13 favors the development of TH2 allergic diseases (e.g. asthma, allergic rhinitis). Certain polymorphisms in the IL-13 gene generate susceptibility to these allergies.

Anti-IL-13 monoclonal antibodies (e.g. Lebrikizumab and Tralokinumab) could be useful to treat TH2 allergies. These drugs are especially useful in patients with high levels of serum periostin (biomarker of IL-13 activity).

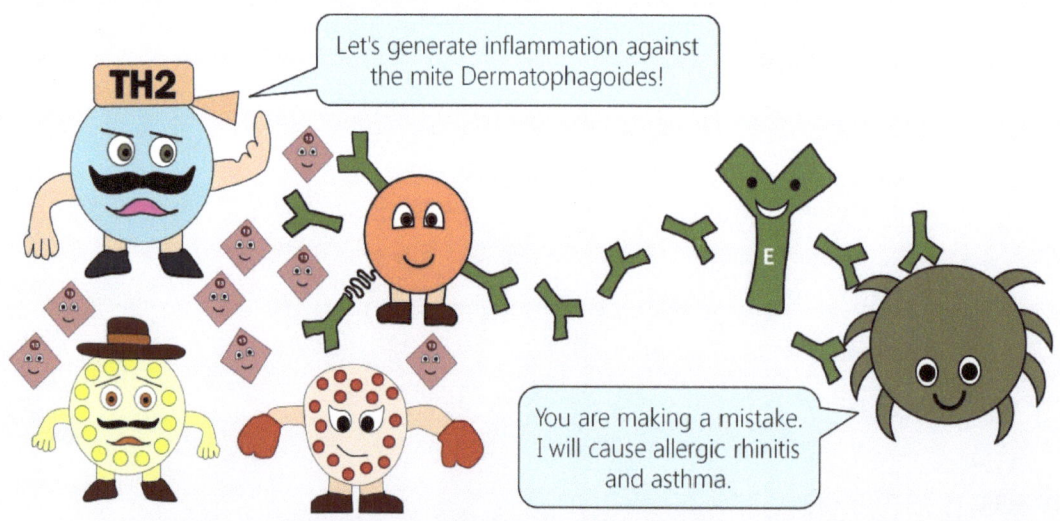

Iris, the interleukin 14

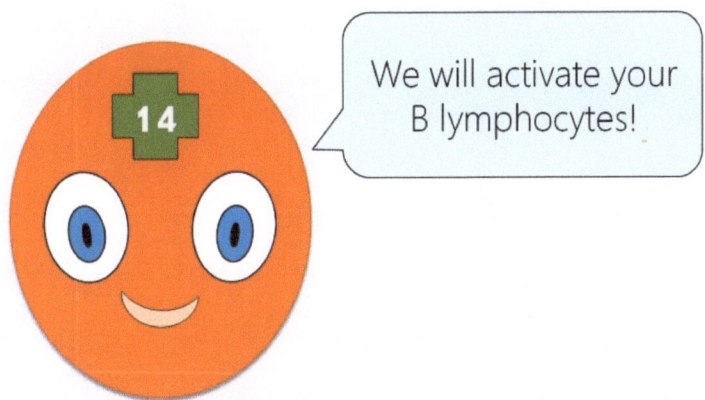

Interleukin 14 is also known as alpha-taxilin or high molecular weight B-cell growth factor (HMW-BCGF). Its receptor is expressed primarily in activated B lymphocytes.

Where is Iris produced?

The main sources of IL-14 are T lymphocytes and some tumor clones of T and B cells.

The main function of Iris is to induce the proliferation of activated B lymphocytes.

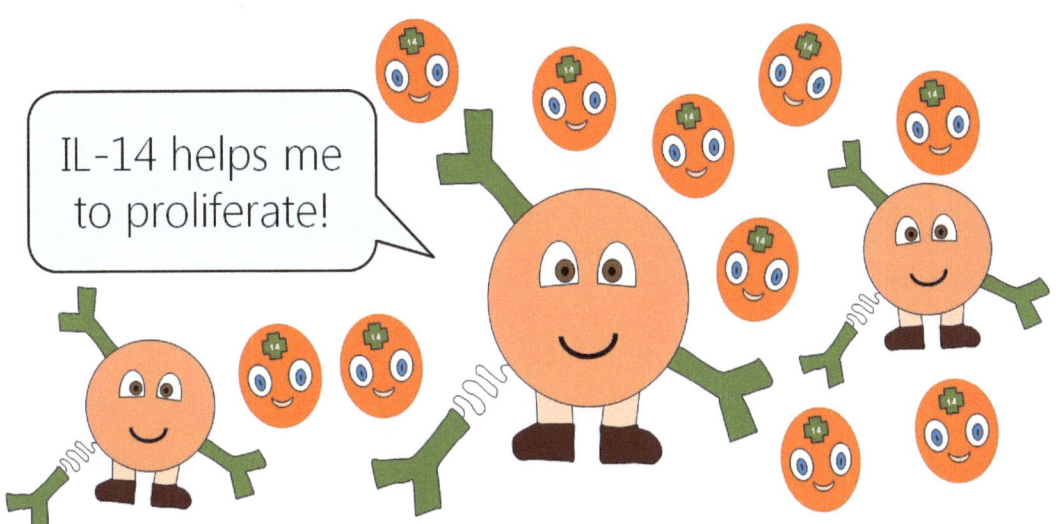

Are there people who cannot produce IL-14?

To date, no human immunodeficiencies have been reported due to the absence of IL-14

Are there people who fabricate IL-14 in excess?

IL-14 favors the proliferation of B lymphocytes, which could be useful to fight against infections.

However, the activity of IL-14 becomes dangerous if activated B lymphocytes are:

- Malignant, capable of inducing B cell neoplasms (e.g. B lymphomas).

- Self-reactive, capable of generating autoimmune diseases by autoantibody production (e.g. systemic lupus erythematosus, Sjögren's syndrome, rheumatoid arthritis, etc.).

Could IL-14 be a therapeutic target in patients with B-cell neoplasms or autoimmunity? We do not know yet, but it is an interesting hypothesis that could be investigated.

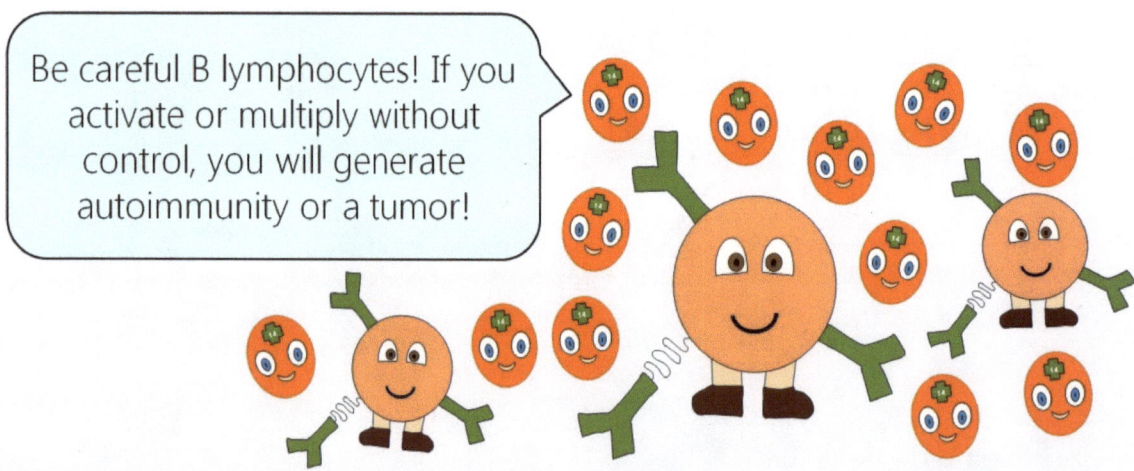

Vicki, the interleukin 15

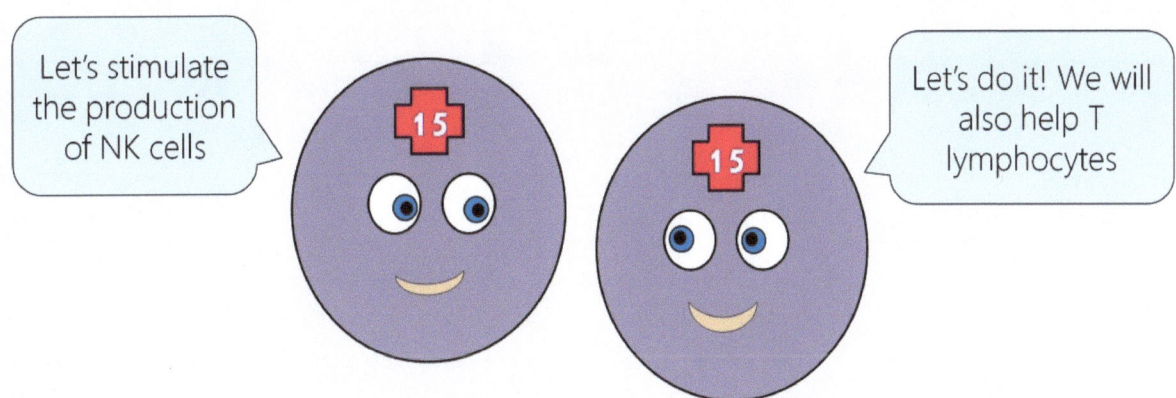

IL-15 exerts similar actions to IL-2 (they are structurally similar), although with greater influence in the production of NK lymphocytes.

The receptor of Vicki, our IL-15, consists of 3 subunits: IL-15Rα, IL-2Rβ and the common gamma chain (γc). Do not forget that γc is also part of the receptors of interleukins 2, 4, 7, 9 and 21.

Where is Vicki produced?

Many cells are capable of making IL-15, including monocytes/macrophages, dendritic cells, activated T CD4 lymphocytes, keratinocytes, skeletal muscle cells, fibroblasts, epithelial cells, bone marrow stromal cells and nerve cells.

The major role of IL-15 is to induce the production and activation of NK lymphocytes. It also activates T lymphocytes and innate lymphoid cells. Furthermore, it promotes the survival of neutrophils and eosinophils.

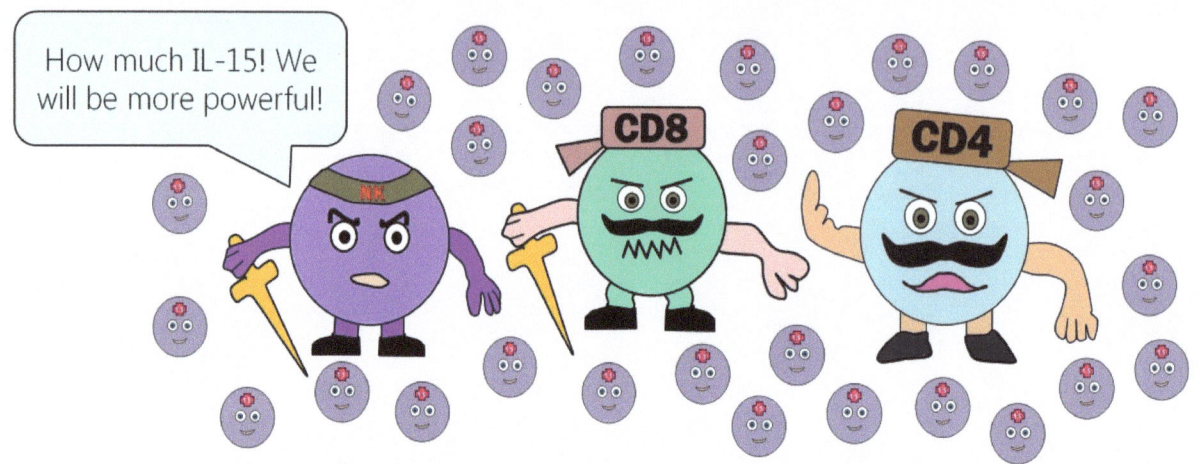

Are there people who cannot produce IL-15?

Children lacking γc have severe X-linked combined immunodeficiency. They cannot produce T or NK lymphocytes because signaling of interleukins 2, 7 and 15 is abolished.

Human recombinant IL-15 may help patients with neoplasms and immunodeficiencies by potentiating T and NK lymphocytes.

Are there people who fabricate IL-15 in excess?

Excessive activity of IL-15 may favor the development of autoimmune diseases (e.g. type 1 diabetes, systemic lupus erythematosus, sarcoidosis, pemphigus, rheumatoid arthritis, celiac disease, psoriasis, etc.). In patients with these diseases the use of anti-IL-15 monoclonal antibodies might be useful.

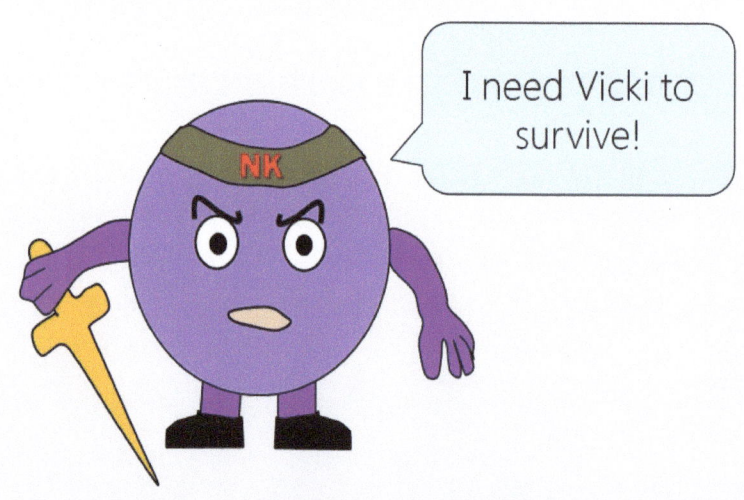

Jess, the interleukin 16

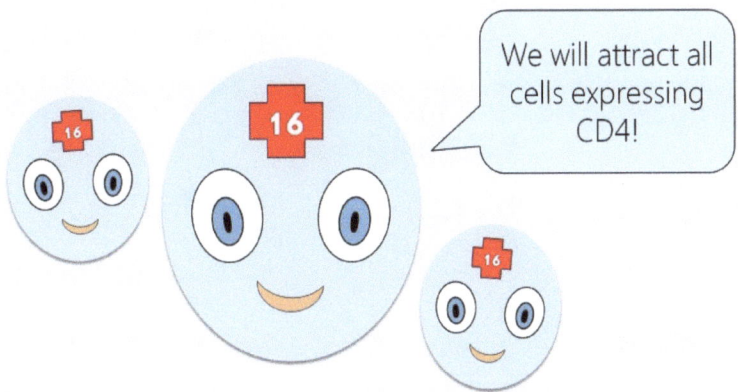

Jess is a cytokine with chemotactic activity. Its receptor is the CD4 protein, so, Jess attracts cells expressing this molecule (e.g. T CD4 lymphocytes, monocytes/macrophages, dendritic cells, mast cells, eosinophils).

Jess was also called 'lymphocyte chemoattractant factor'.

Where is Jess produced?

Cells that produce IL-16 include T lymphocytes, eosinophils, mast cells, monocytes, dendritic cells, epithelial cells and fibroblasts. Jess is synthesized when caspase 3 cleaves the precursor pro-IL-16.

In addition to its chemotactic ability, Jess modulates the action of T lymphocytes:

- Promotes TH1 immunity by activating secretion of TNF-α, IL-1β and IL-15.

- Reduces TH2 inflammation by inhibiting the synthesis of IL-4 and IL-5.

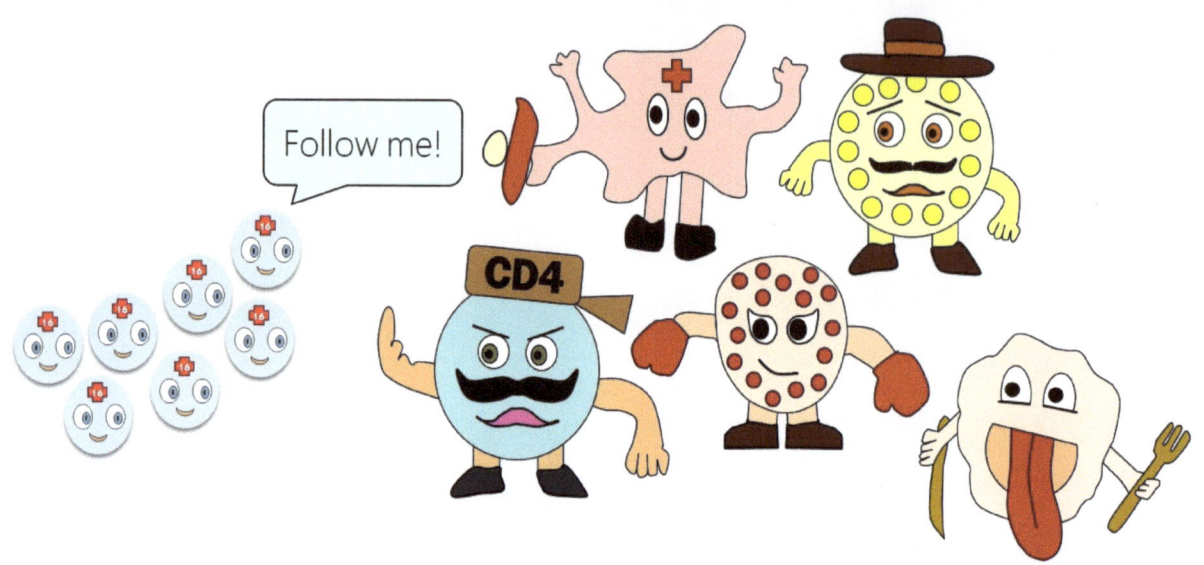

Are there people who cannot produce IL-16?

Immunodeficiencies caused by genetic defects of IL-16 have not been described yet.

¿Hay personas que fabrican IL-16 en exceso o inapropiadamente?

Polymorphisms in the IL-16 gene that increase the activity of this cytokine may favor the development of inflammatory diseases (e.g. rheumatoid arthritis, endometriosis, reperfusion injury, multiple sclerosis, chronic hepatitis B, transplant rejection, cancer).

IL-16 serum levels could be a biomarker of activity in these diseases. Moreover, affected patients could benefit from the use of anti-IL-16 antibodies.

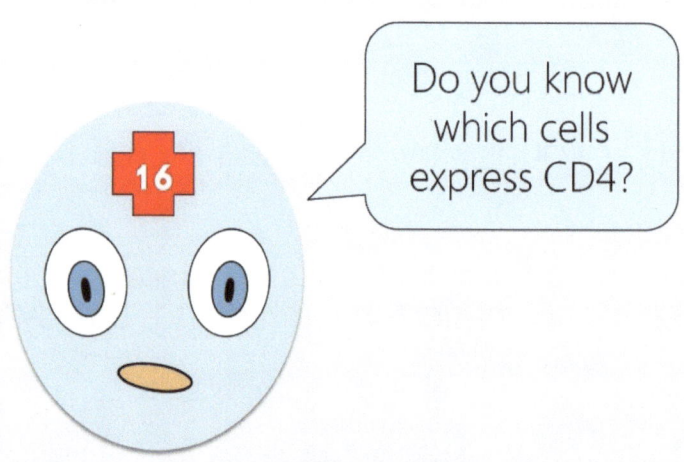

Anne, the IL-17A, and her sisters

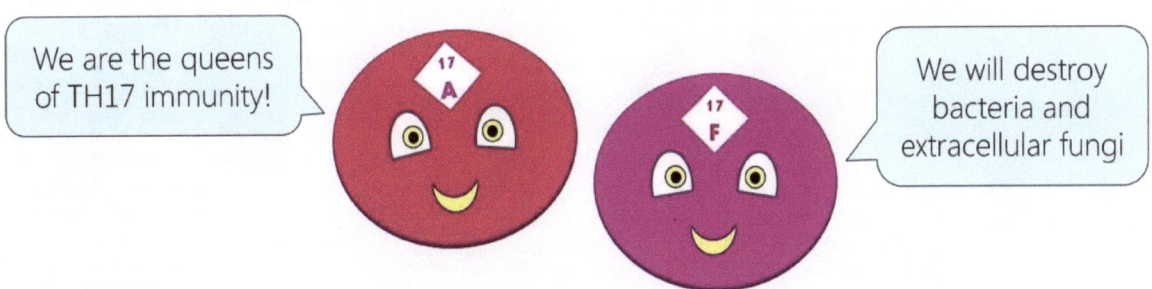

The interleukin 17 family has 6 members: IL-17A, IL-17B, IL-17C, IL-17D, IL-17E (also named IL-25) and IL-17F.

Anne is our powerful IL-17A. She acts through IL-17RA receptor to protect us from the attack of extracellular fungi and bacteria (e.g. *Candida albicans*, *Staphylococcus aureus*). The same functions are fulfilled by her sister Ana, our IL-17F, through its receptor formed by the subunits IL-17RA and IL-17RC.

Where are they produced?

Anne and Ana are mainly produced by TH17 lymphocytes and type 3 innate lymphoid cells. Both have proinflammatory actions:

- Activation of epithelial cells to synthesize antimicrobial peptides and chemokines.

- Recruitment and activation of neutrophils.

Are there people who cannot produce IL-17A or IL-17F?

Patients with pathogenic mutations in the IL-17F, IL-17RA or IL-17RC genes are susceptible to infections by extracellular fungi and bacteria, especially *Candida albicans*.

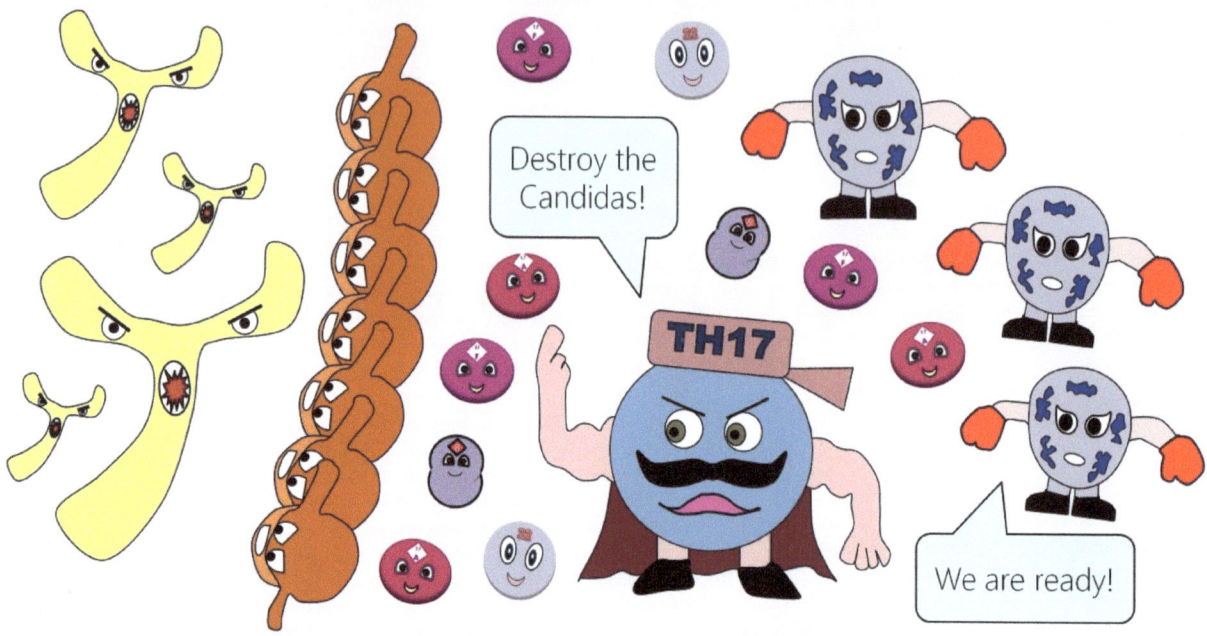

The same problem affects patients with genetic defects that impede the development of TH17 lymphocytes (e.g. CARD9, STAT3 or ACT1 deficiencies, STAT1 hyperfunction).

Are there people who fabricate IL-17A or IL-17F in excess?

Several autoimmune diseases (e.g. rheumatoid arthritis, psoriasis, neutrophilic asthma) occur due to a pathologic activity of our TH17 army with excessive production of IL-17A and IL-17F. Affected patients may improve with drugs targeting these cytokines, such as:

- Secukinumab and Ixekizumab (anti-IL-17A antibodies).

- Bimekizumab (dual inhibitor of IL-17A and IL-17F) or Brodalumab (anti-IL-17RA monoclonal antibody).

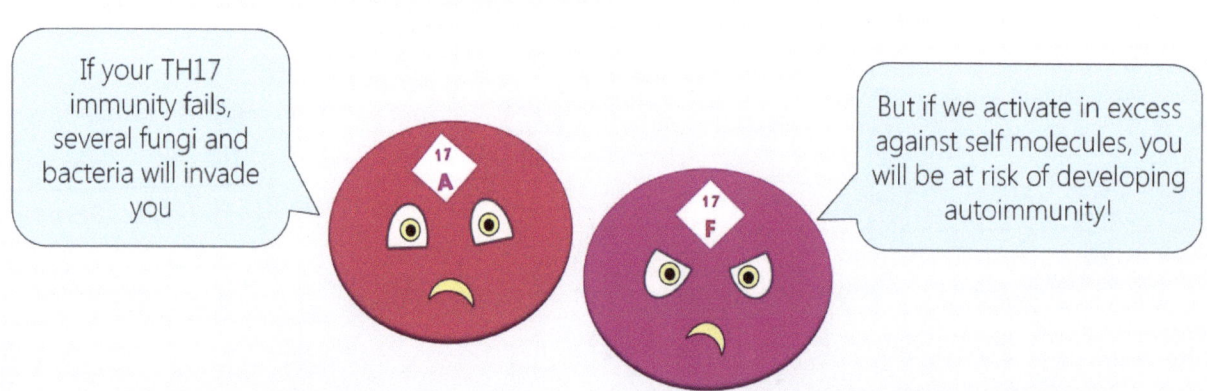

Pia, the interleukin 18

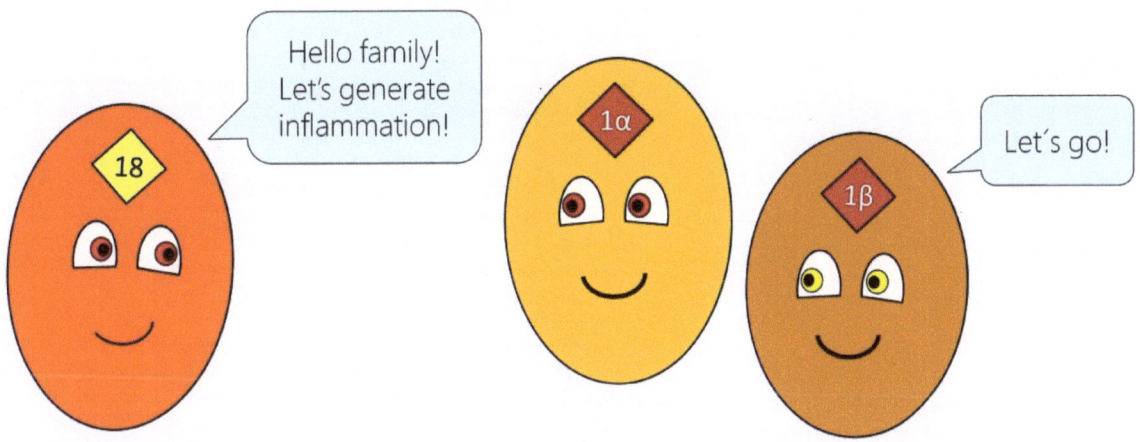

IL-18 belongs to the IL-1 superfamily. It is also called 'interferon-gamma inducing factor'. Its biological activity can be neutralized by IL-18bp (IL-18 binding protein).

Where is Pia produced?

Pia can be synthesized by macrophages, dendritic cells, epithelial cells, chondrocytes and osteoblasts.

The inflammatory action of Pia includes the activation of TH1 and NK cells. Pia induces interferon-γ synthesis and cellular cytotoxicity.

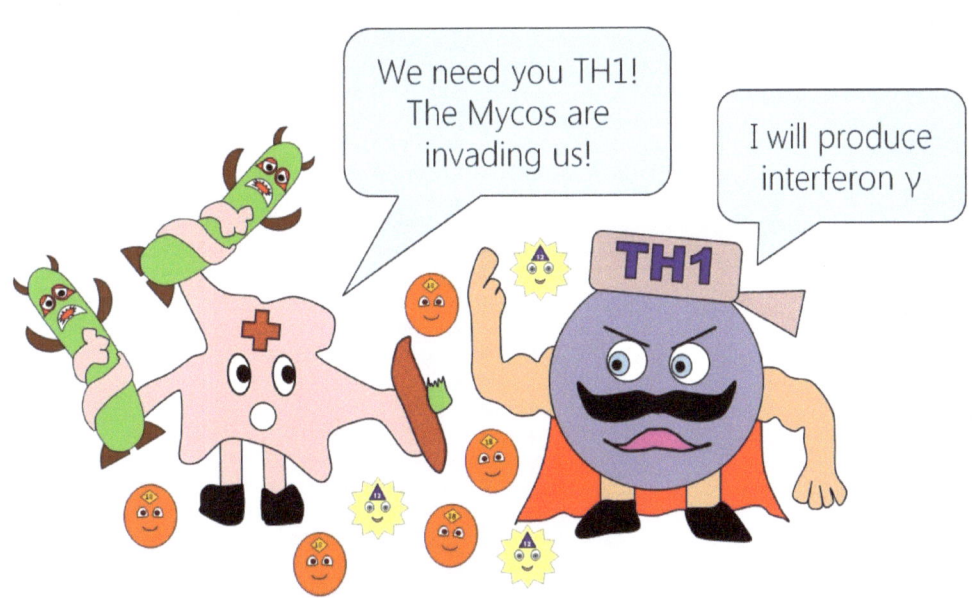

Are there people who cannot produce IL-18?

Human primary immunodeficiencies due to IL-18 gene mutations have not been described yet.

Recombinant human IL-18 could be useful to treat patients with cancer or chronic infections, because of its immune stimulatory activity.

Are there people who fabricate IL-18 in excess?

Yes. Excessive IL-18 production may favor the development of autoimmune and inflammatory diseases (e.g. rheumatoid arthritis, psoriasis, multiple sclerosis, type 1 diabetes, inflammatory bowel disease, Alzheimer's disease, macrophage activation syndrome, hemophagocytosis, autoinflammatory disorders).

In patients with these diseases, IL-18 can be a therapeutic target. For example:

- Tadekinig alfa (human recombinant IL-18bp) is a compound that targets and neutralizes IL-18. Its usefulness has been investigated for the treatment of rheumatoid arthritis, psoriasis and adult-onset Still's disease.

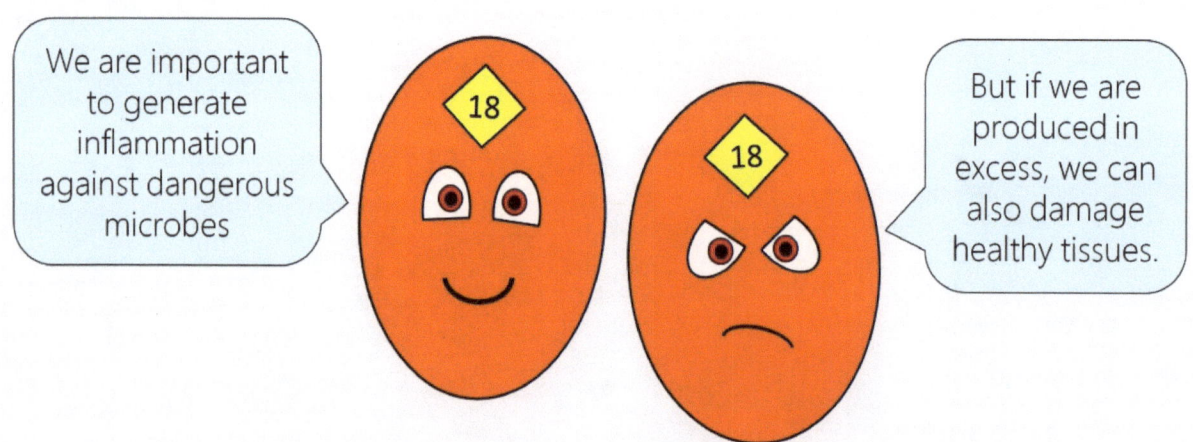

Vane, the interleukin 19

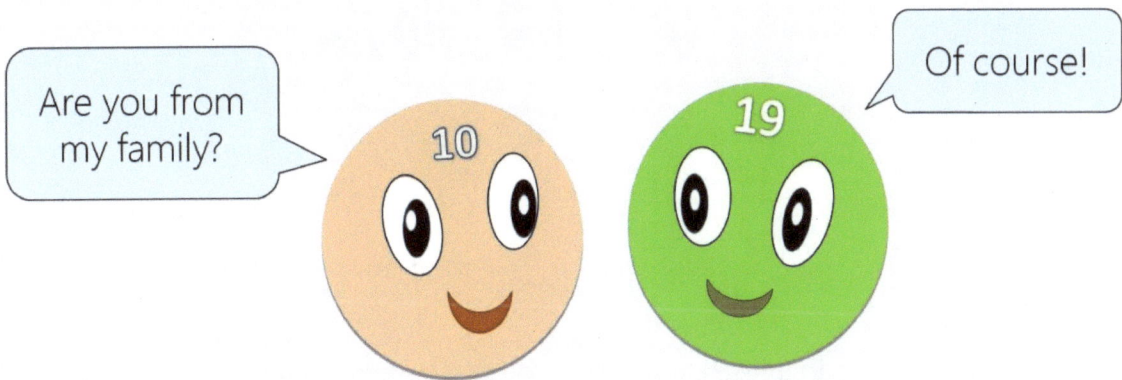

In comparison to other cytokines, there is modest research on IL-19 physiology. Nevertheless, we will review about it.

IL-19 belongs to the interleukin 10 family, along with other cytokines (IL-10, IL-20, IL-22, IL-24, IL-26, IL-28 and IL-29).

However, unlike IL-10 which essentially has regulatory activity, IL-19 can induce the activation of our TH2 army and the proliferation of keratinocytes through its receptor formed by the IL-20R1 and IL-20R2 subunits.

Where is Vane produced?

Vane is produced by various cells, including monocytes, keratinocytes, endothelial cells, epithelial cells and B lymphocytes.

Vane can favor the synthesis of interleukins 4, 5, 10 and 13 from T lymphocytes, thus favoring TH2 immunity. She is also capable of inducing expression of keratinocyte growth factor (KGF).

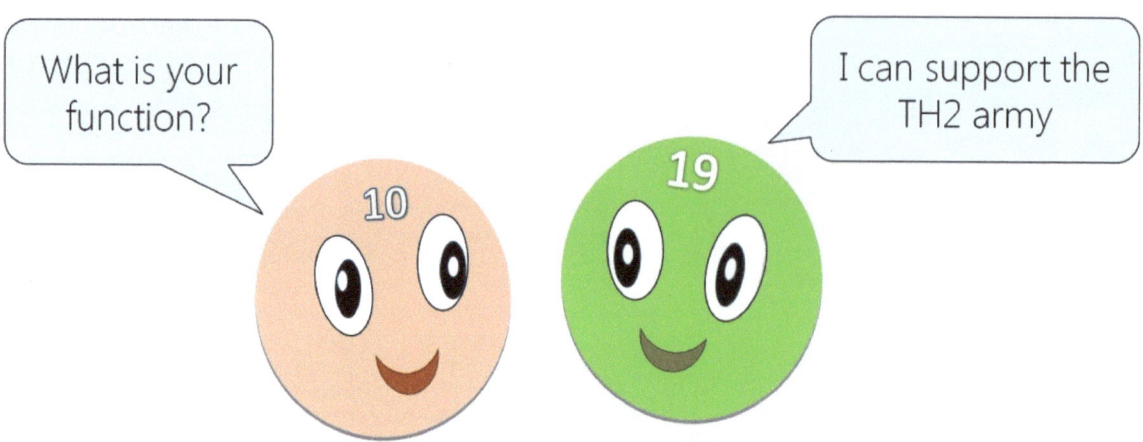

Are there people who cannot produce IL-19?

To the best of our knowledge, there are no reports of people with primary immunodeficiency due to lack of IL-19 synthesis.

Are there people who fabricate IL-19 in excess?

Increased levels of IL-19 have been reported in patients with bronchial asthma. Excessive production of IL-19 could favor the development of TH2 allergic diseases such as asthma or atopic dermatitis.

Moreover, Vane could favor the onset of psoriasis by inducing keratinocyte growth factor (KGF).

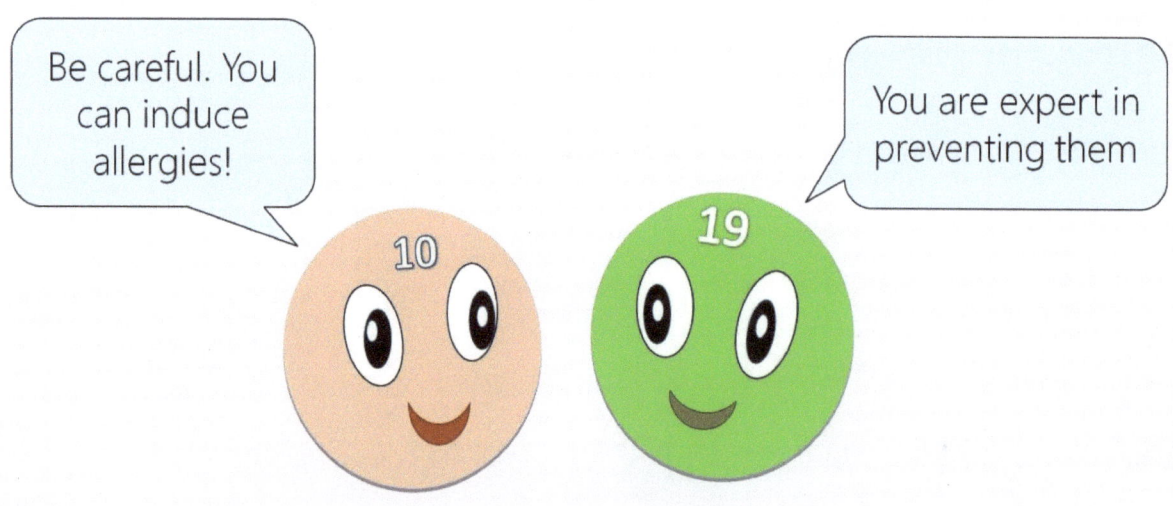

Kate, the interleukin 20

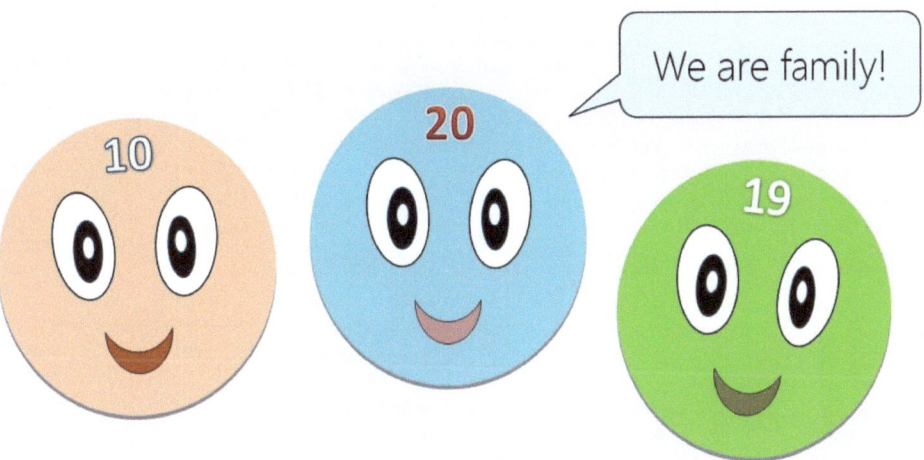

Kate is a member of the interleukin IL-10 family, which includes interleukins 19, 20, 22, 24, 26, 28 and 29. Kate is also recognized as the leader of the interleukin 20 subfamily, together with interleukins 19, 22, 24 and 26, because they share subunits in their respective receptors.

Kate acts through 2 types of receptors: one consists of the IL-20R1 and IL-20R2 subunits; the other is formed by the IL-22R1 and IL-20R2 chains.

Where is Kate produced?

Kate can be synthesized by monocytes, keratinocytes, epithelial cells, dendritic cells and endothelial cells.

Unlike IL-10, Kate is essentially proinflammatory. Her major activity is to induce the proliferation and differentiation of epithelial cells during inflammatory processes, especially in the skin. She can also favor the expansion of multipotent hematopoietic progenitor cells.

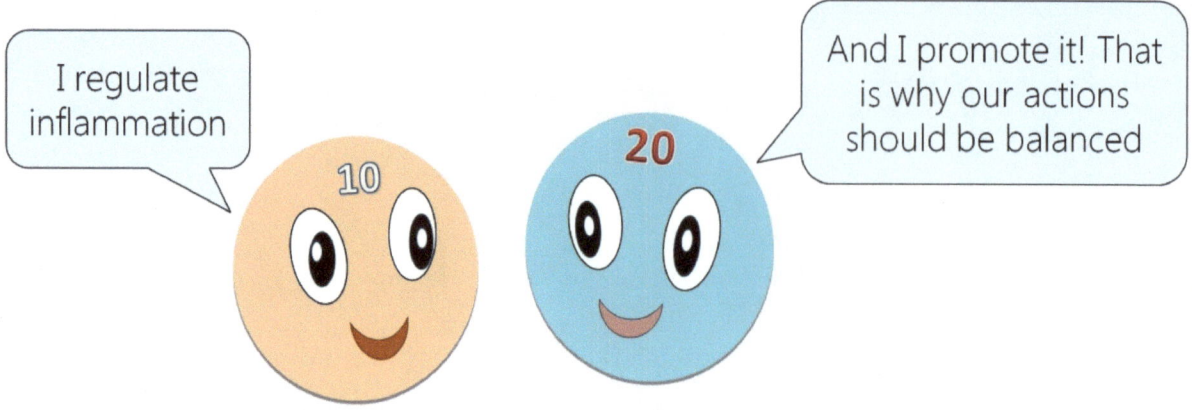

Are there people who cannot produce IL-20?

To date, no individuals with inherited errors of IL-20 production have been reported.

Are there people who fabricate IL-20 in excess?

Similar to interleukin 19, IL-20 may have an inductive role in the pathogenesis of psoriasis.

In addition, an excess of IL-20 activity has been reported in other inflammatory diseases (asthma, rheumatoid arthritis, systemic lupus erythematosus, obesity, atherosclerosis, ulcerative colitis, osteoporosis, multiple myeloma).

For this reason, IL-20 can represent a biomarker of disease activity and a therapeutic target in affected patients.

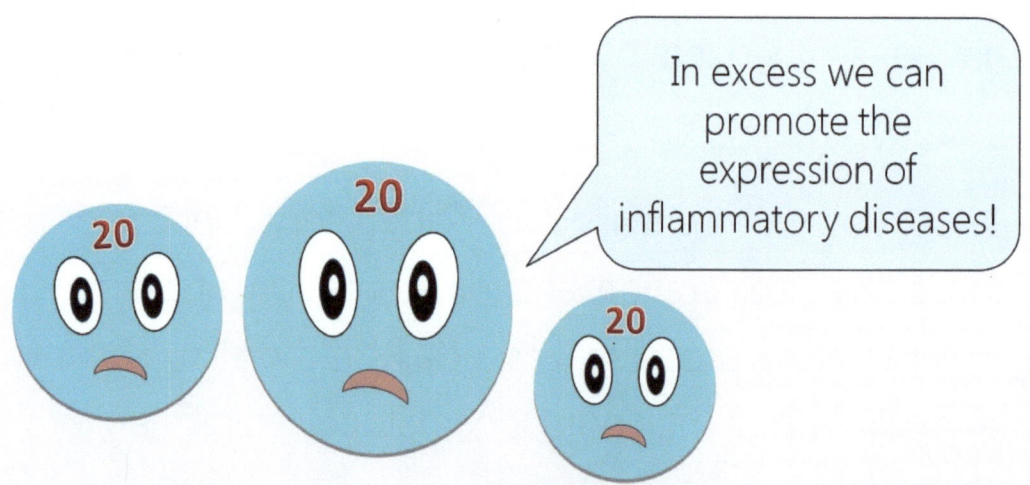

Lisa, the interleukin 21

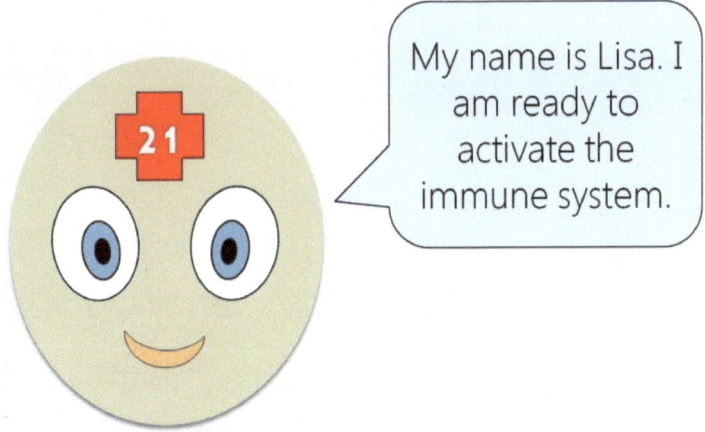

Lisa exerts her immune-stimulating actions through the IL-21R receptor, which is made up of the IL-21Rα subunit and the common gamma chain (γc). Remember that γc is also part of the receptors of interleukins 2, 4, 7, 9 and 15.

Where is Lisa produced?

The main source of IL-21 are T lymphocytes, mainly follicular helper T cells, which potentiate B lymphocytes in the follicles of secondary lymphatic organs such as lymph nodes and spleen. Other sources of IL-21 are TH2, TH9, TH17 and NKT lymphocytes.

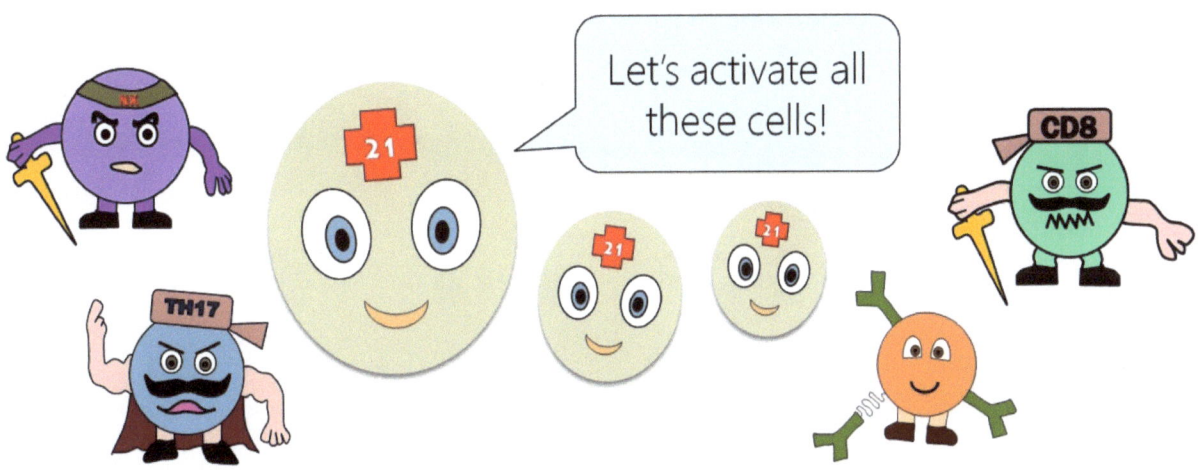

Lisa is able to stimulate:

- Proliferation, specialization and maturation of B lymphocytes.
- Cytotoxic activity of CD8 and NKT lymphocytes.
- Activation of TH17 lymphocytes.

Are there people who cannot produce IL-21?

X-linked severe combined immunodeficiency (X-SCID) occurs due to pathogenic mutations in the γc gene. Patients with X-SCID are fragile against all types of microbes because the signaling of interleukins 2, 4, 7, 9, 15 and 21 is impaired.

Recombinant human IL-21 (Denenicokin) is a potential therapy against neoplasms and chronic viral infections by potentiating CD8 and NKT lymphocytes.

Are there people who fabricate IL-21 in excess?

Overproduction of IL-21 after recognition of self molecules favors the development of autoimmune diseases (e.g. systemic lupus erythematosus, rheumatoid arthritis, psoriasis, type 1 diabetes). Anti-IL-21 monoclonal antibodies may have a therapeutic role in these diseases.

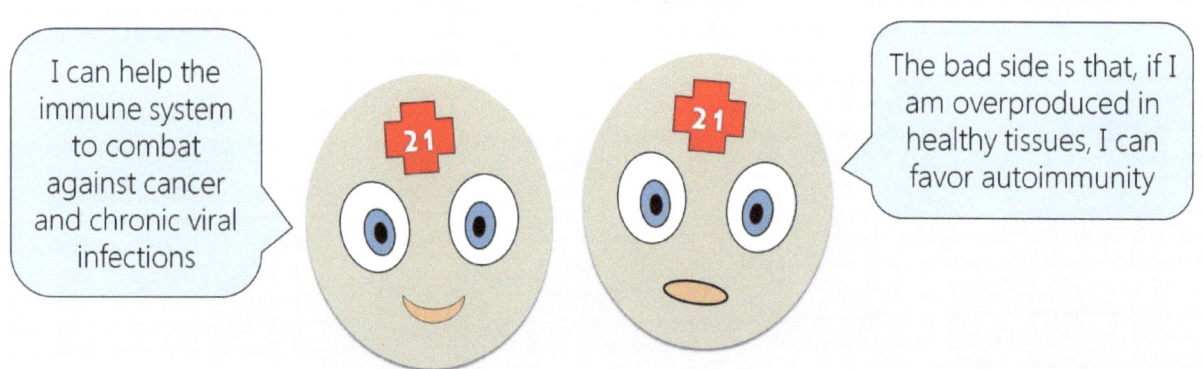

Sami, the interleukin 22

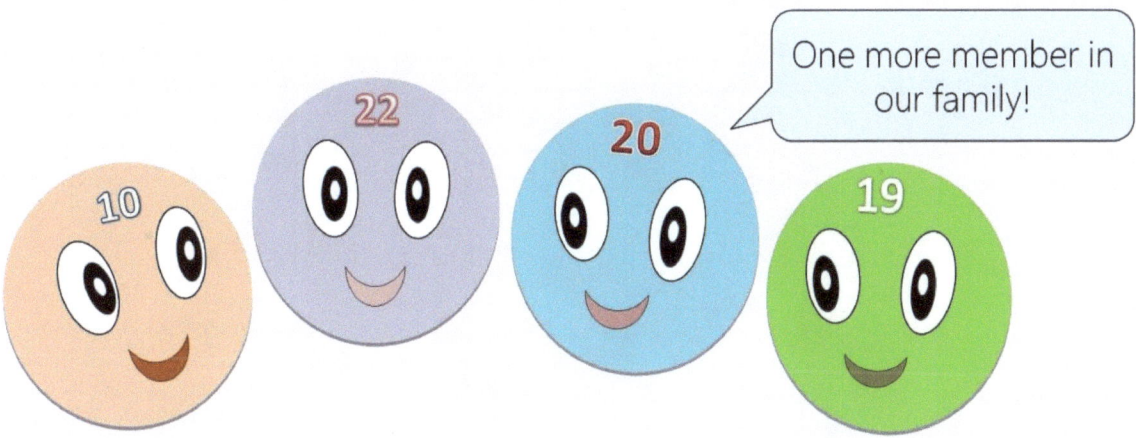

Our wonderful Sami belongs to the family of IL-10 and the subfamily of IL-20. Its receptor is made up of the IL-22R1 and IL-10R2 chains.

A differential feature of Sami among cytokines is that she is produced by immune cells but acts on non-hematopoietic stromal cells.

Where is Sami produced?

Sami can be synthesized by several types of cells: TH22 lymphocytes, TH17 lymphocytes, type 3 innate lymphoid cells, lymphoid tissue inducer cells, mast cells and NK lymphocytes.

The main target cells of IL-22 are keratinocytes and epithelial cells of the kidney, gut, liver, pancreas and lung.

Sami promotes innate defense against pathogenic microbes, synthesis of antimicrobial peptides (e.g. defensins), cell proliferation and tissue repair.

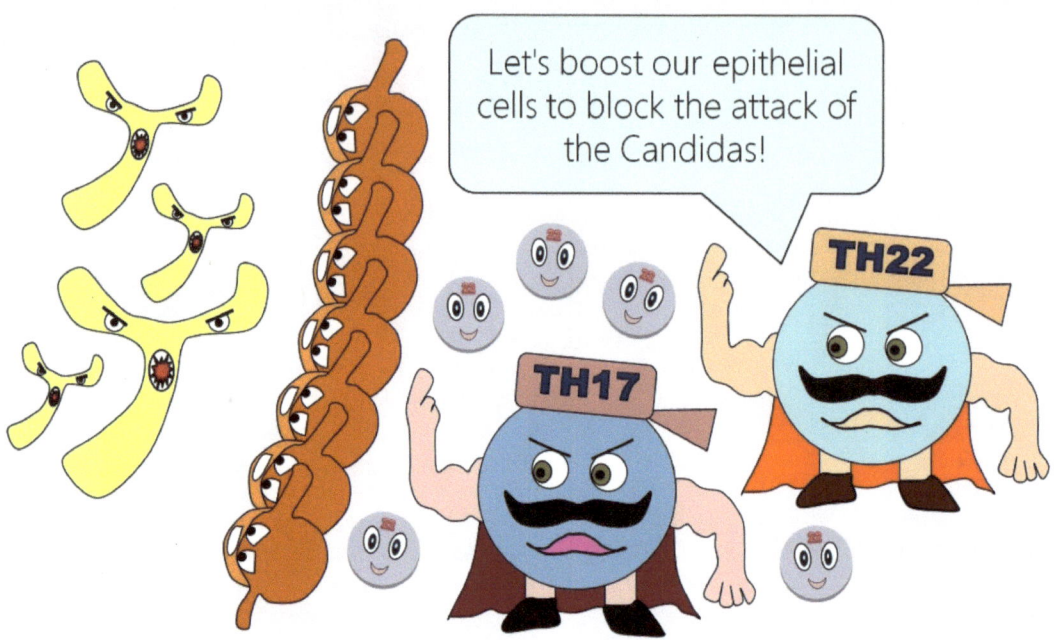

Are there people who cannot produce IL-22?

Patients with genetic defects affecting TH17 immunity (e.g. STAT1 hyperfunction, CARD9 deficiency) are less able to produce IL-22. As a consequence, innate defense in skin and mucosas is weakened, thereby increasing the risk of fungal and bacterial infections.

Are there people who fabricate IL-22 in excess?

Patients with psoriasis and atopic dermatitis have increased IL-22 levels in the skin. By inducing proliferation of epithelial cells, excess IL-22 can promote the appearance of epithelial neoplasms and inflammatory diseases such as rheumatoid arthritis.

Fezakinumab (anti-IL-22) could not reach commercialization.

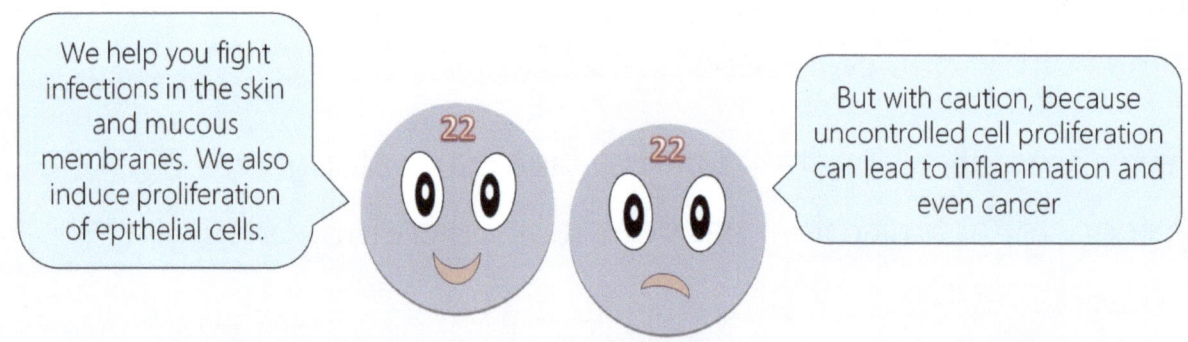

Mari, the interleukin 23

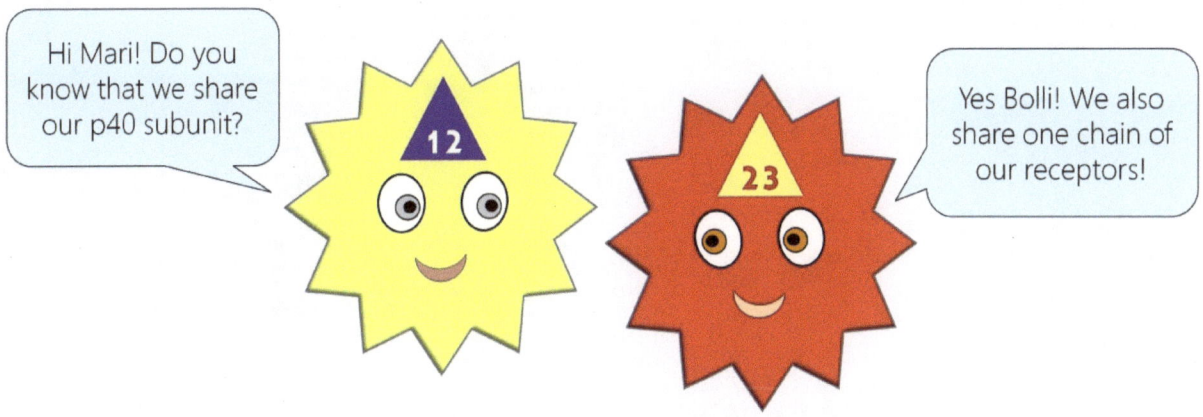

Mari has 2 subunits: IL-23p19 and IL-12p40. Remind that IL-12p40 is also part of Bolli, our interleukin 12.

The receptor of IL-23 is composed of 2 chains: IL-12Rβ1 (it also makes up the IL-12 receptor) and IL-23R.

Where is Mari produced?

Mari is mainly produced by dendritic cells and macrophages in response to the attack of extracellular bacteria and fungi (e.g. *Candida albicans, Staphylococcus aureus*). Mari is an essential component in the fight against these microbes by inducing the differentiation of our TH17 lymphocytes.

Are there people who cannot produce IL-23?

Individuals with genetic deficiencies of the IL-12p40 subunit or the IL-12Rβ1 chain have impaired signaling of interleukins 12 and 23, becoming susceptible to infections by several microbes, both intracellular (e.g. mycobacteria, *Salmonella spp, Histoplasma capsulatum*) and extracellular (e.g. *Candida albicans*).

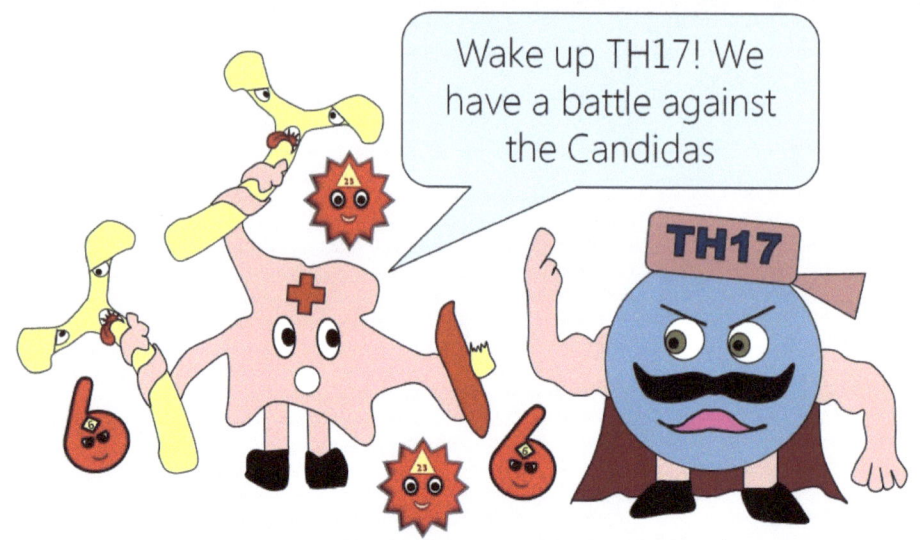

Are there people who fabricate IL-23 in excess?

Excessive production of IL-23 against self molecules promotes the appearance of inflammatory diseases, such as psoriasis, Crohn's disease, spondyloarthropathies and lupus. Affected patients may benefit from IL-23 inhibition. For example:

- The monoclonal antibodies Guselkumab and Tildrakizumab are directed against the subunit IL-23p19, thus inhibiting the activity of the TH17 immune army.

- The biological drug Ustekinumab neutralizes the IL-12p40 subunit of interleukins 12 and 23. In consequence, it exerts an inhibitory effect on both TH1 and TH17 armies.

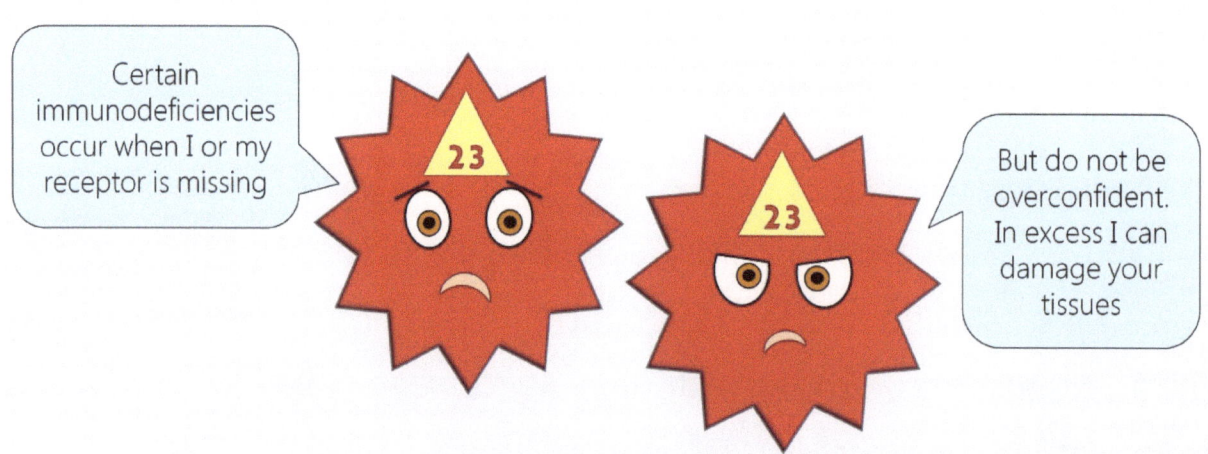

Lila, the interleukin 24

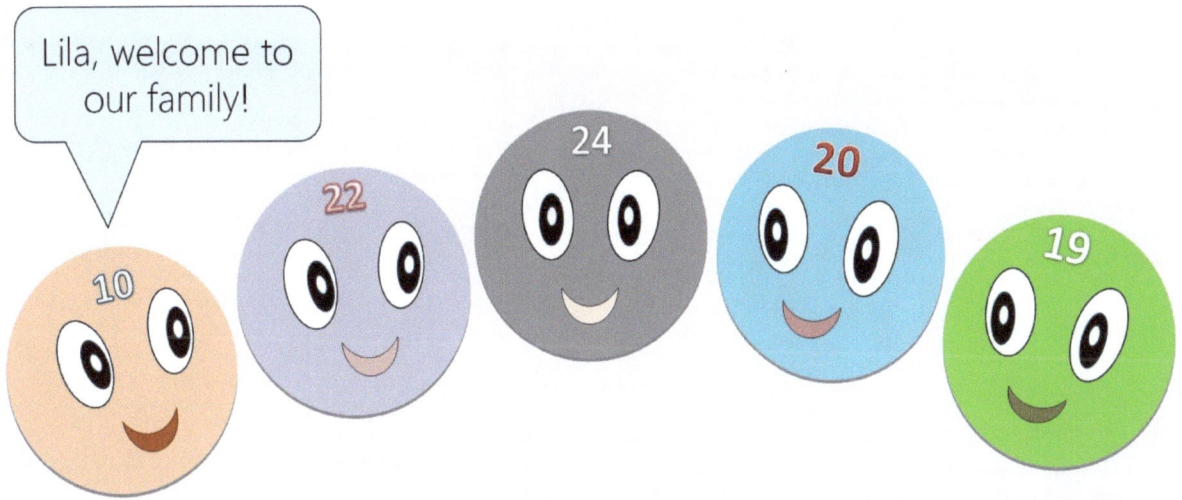

Lila, also called MDA-7 (melanoma differentiation associated gene-7), belongs to the IL-10 family and the IL-20 subfamily. It performs its functions through 2 receptors: IL-20R1/IL-20R2 and IL-22R1/IL-20R2.

Lila loves to inhibit the growth of malignant cancer cells.

Where is Lila produced?

Lila can be synthesized by hematopoietic cells (e.g. monocytes, T lymphocytes, B cells) and non-hematopoietic cells (e.g. melanocytes, keratinocytes). She has diverse biological functions related to cell proliferation, differentiation and apoptosis. However, its most recognized ability is to block the proliferation of tumor cells.

Recent research has shown that IL-24 might have inhibitory activity against influenza virus.

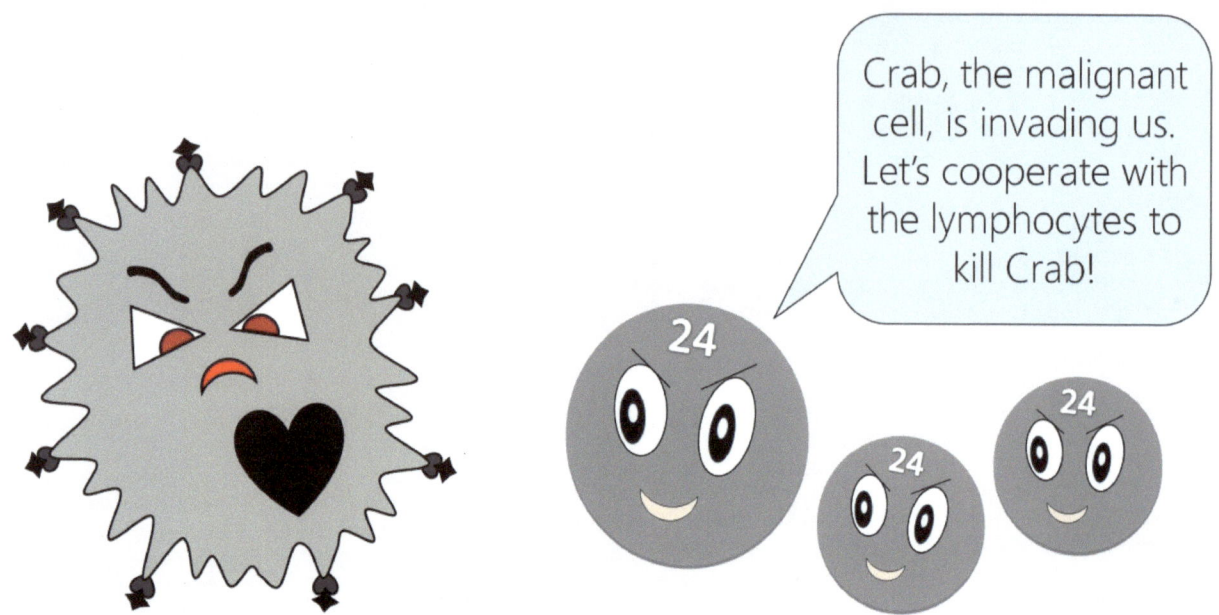

Are there people who cannot produce IL-24?

Primary immunodeficiencies due to mutations in the IL-24 gene have not been reported.

Therapy with recombinant IL-24 has the potential to inhibit the growth of malignant cells in patients with cancer.

Are there people who fabricate IL-24 in excess?

Excessive synthesis of IL-24 could favor the onset of inflammatory diseases such as psoriasis.

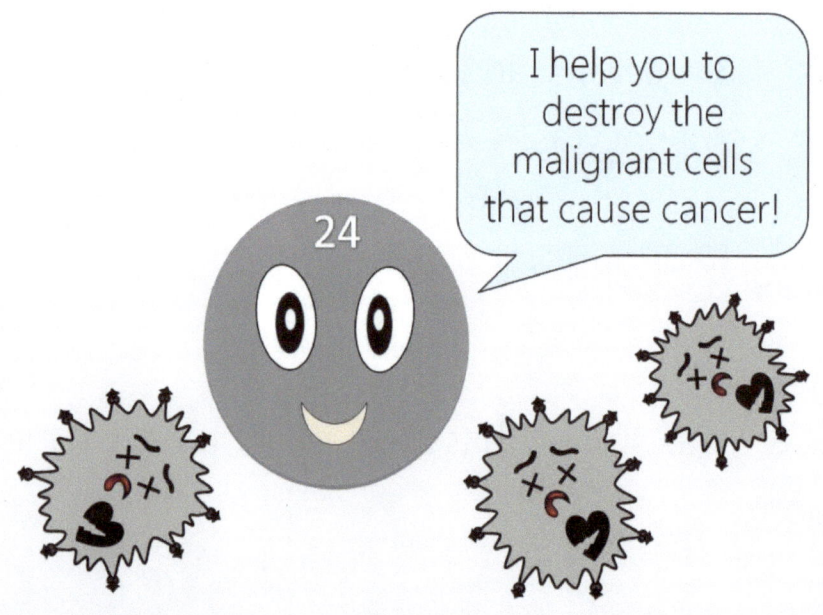

Flor, the interleukin 25

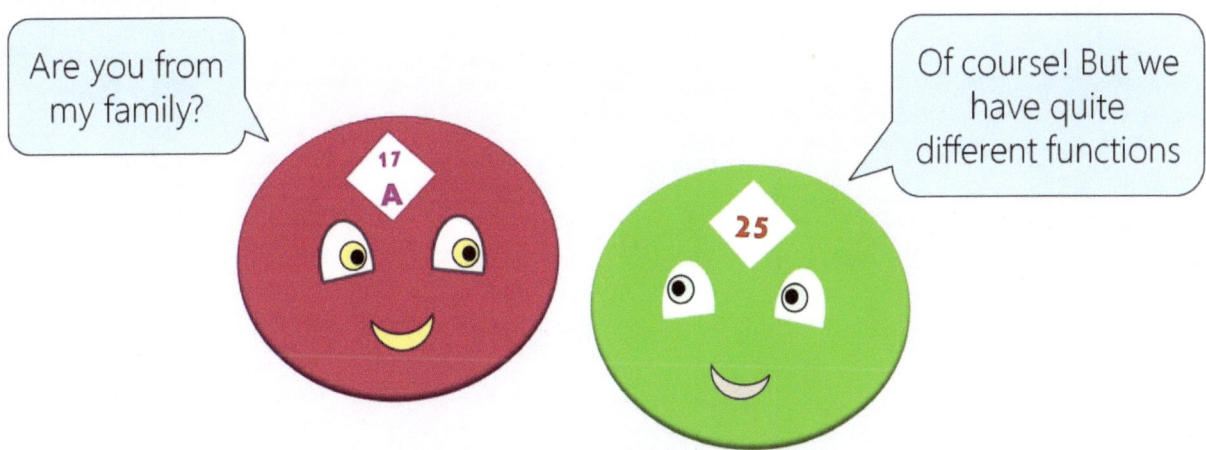

Flor, also known as IL-17E, is a member of the interleukin 17 family. However, unlike her sisters IL-17A and IL-17F, Flor is a cytokine that activates our TH2 army. Her receptor has 2 chains: IL-17RA and IL-17RB.

Where is Flor produced?

Flor is made by epithelial cells and several cells of the TH2 army (TH2 lymphocytes, eosinophils, mast cells and basophils).

Flor activates our TH2 army in the battle against helminths, by promoting synthesis of IgE and interleukins 4, 5, 9 and 13.

It is very interesting to note that, like IL-24, Flor has the ability to destroy malignant cells that cause cancer.

Are there people who cannot produce IL-25?

IL-25-deficient mice are less able to expel the helminth *Nippostrongylus brasiliensis*.

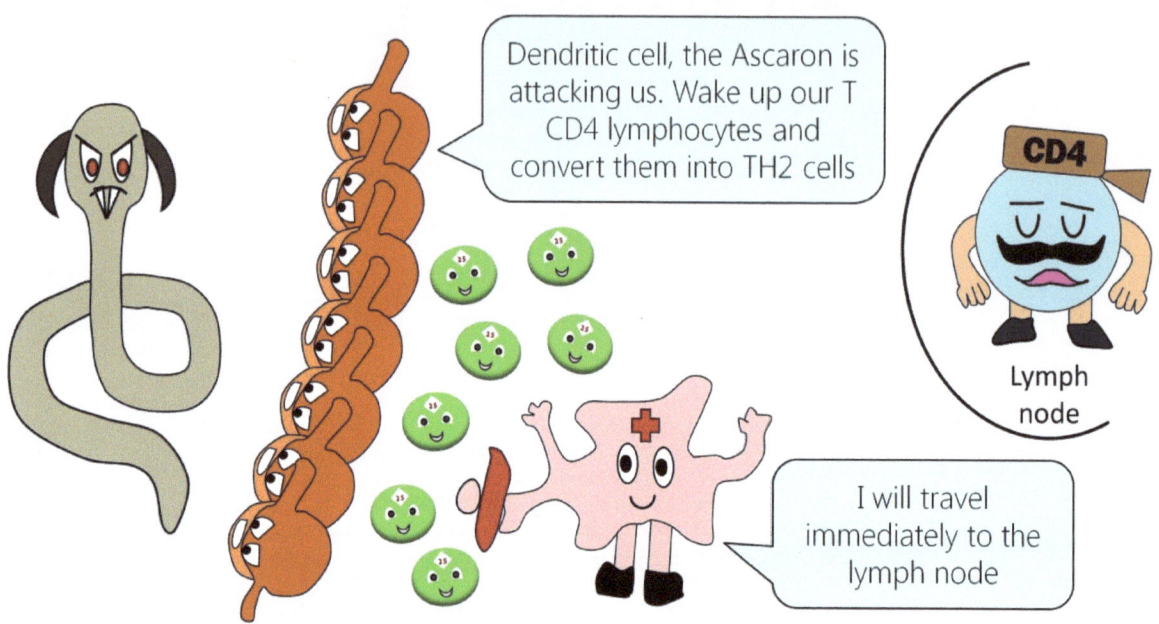

Patients with genetic mutations in *IL17RA* are susceptible to extracellular fungal and bacterial infections, because of impaired signaling of IL-17A and IL-17F.

IL-25 is a potential treatment for cancer.

Are there people who fabricate IL-25 in excess?

Excessive production of IL-25 after exposure to beneficial or harmless molecules (e.g. *Dermatophagoides* mites) induces the development of TH2 allergies (e.g. asthma, allergic rhinitis). Affected patients may benefit from anti-IL-25 biological therapies.

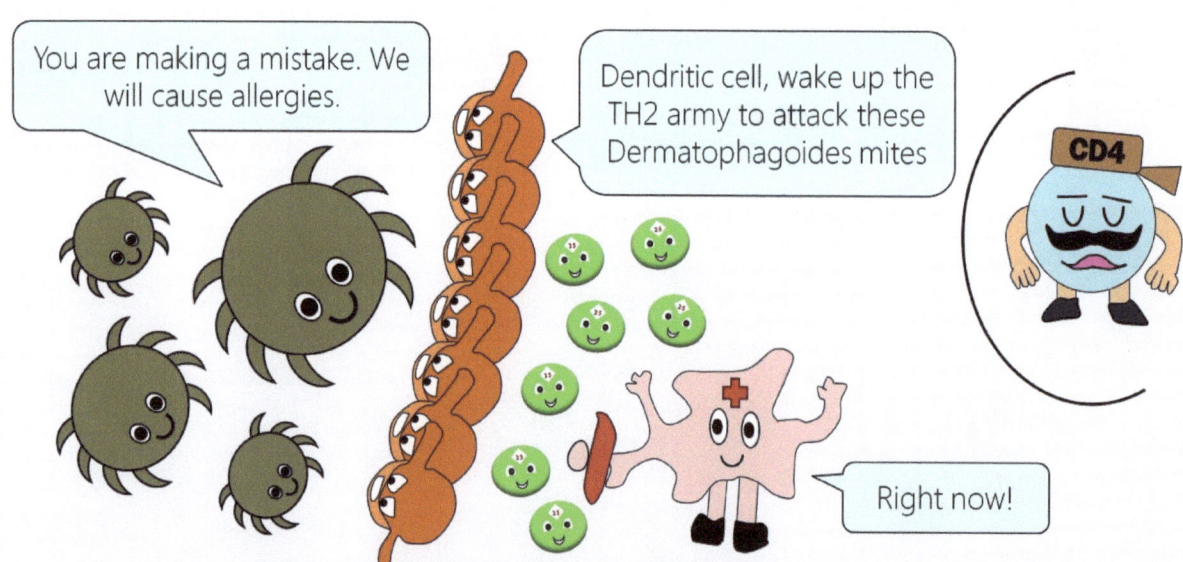

Shen, the interleukin 26

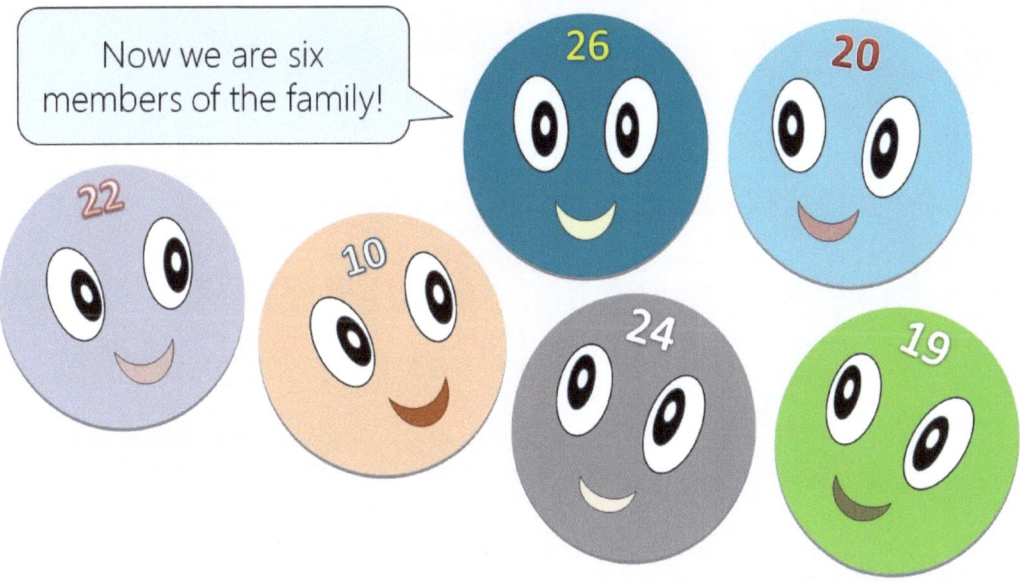

Shen is part of the IL-10 family and the IL-20 subfamily. Her receptor consists of two chains: IL-10R2 and IL-20R1.

Where is Shen produced?

Cells that produce IL-26 include T lymphocytes, especially TH17 cells, and NK lymphocytes.

Shen has several antimicrobial actions:

- Promotes the secretion of proinflammatory cytokines IL-1β, IL-8 and TNF-α. Do not forget that IL-8 attracts neutrophils.

- Destroys extracellular bacteria through membrane pores.

- Participates in the recognition of microbial DNA.

- Promotes antiviral defense by stimulating interferon production.

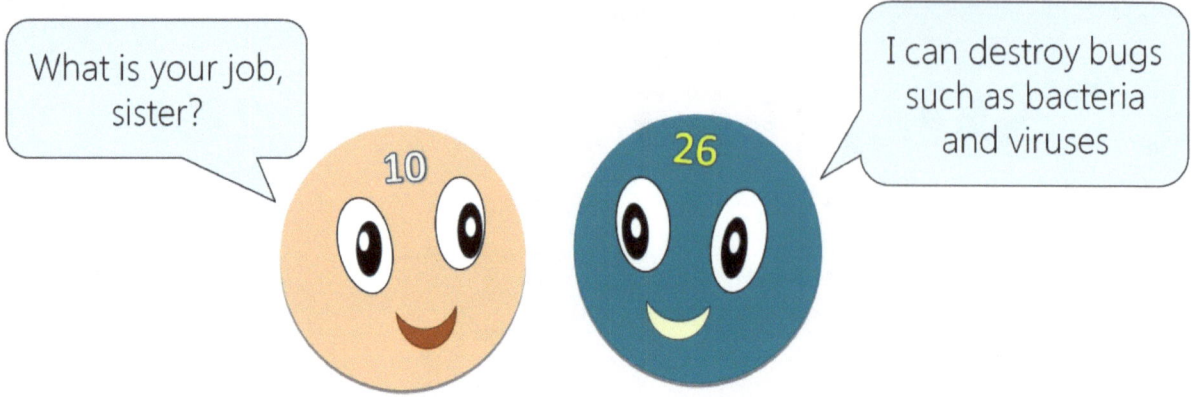

Are there people who cannot produce IL-26?

Children with genetic defects in IL-10 receptor (IL-10R1 or IL-10R2) develop severe early-onset inflammatory diseases (inflammatory bowel disease with perianal fistulas, folliculitis, arthritis) secondary to impaired IL-10 signaling.

IL-26 could be useful to prevent osteoclast-induced bone lysis.

Are there people who fabricate IL-26 in excess?

TH17-derived interleukin 26 can promote the development of Crohn's disease, rheumatoid arthritis and multiple sclerosis. Therapies targeting TH17 immunity are useful in patients with these autoimmune diseases.

Shen might be useful as a biomarker for neutrophilic diseases such as non-TH2-mediated asthma.

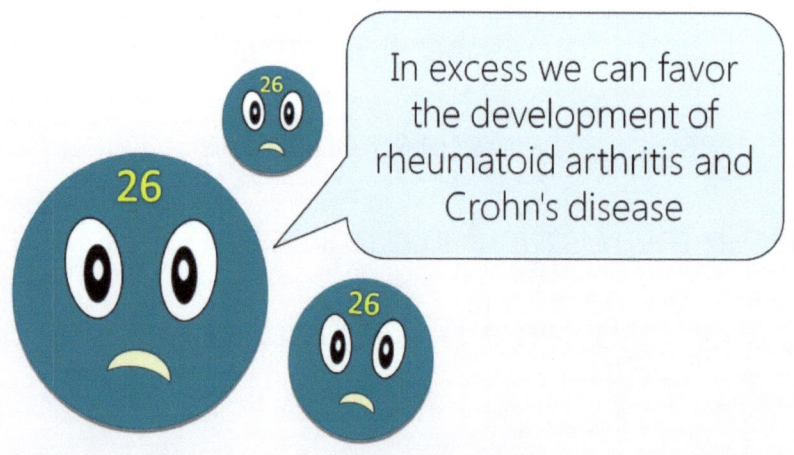

Luna, the interleukin 27

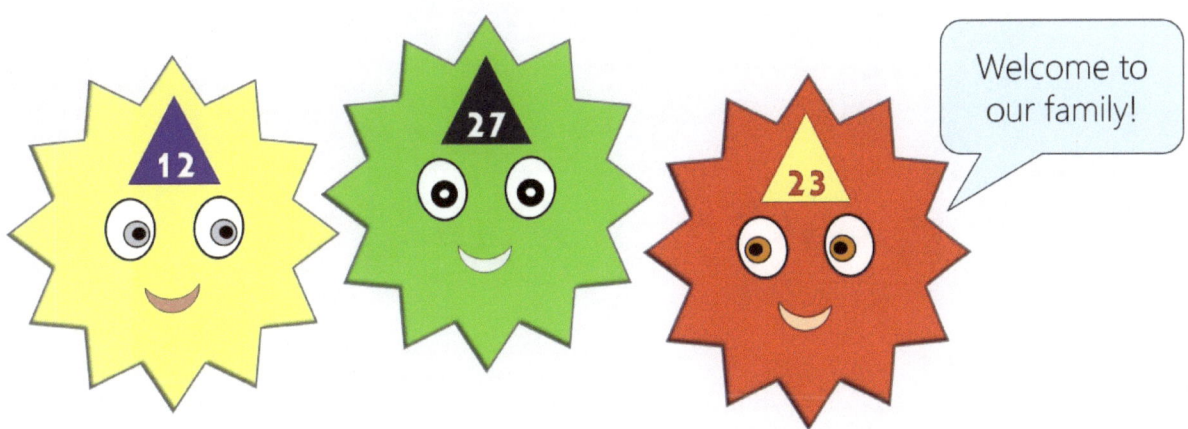

Luna, nuestra hermosa interleucina 27, es parte de la familia de la IL-12. Tiene 2 subunidades: p28 (¡esta subunidad es la IL-30!) y EBI-3. Su receptor consta de 2 cadenas: gp130 (también forma parte de los receptores de IL-6, IL-11 e IL-35) e IL-27Rα.

Where is Luna produced?

Luna, que puede ser fabricada por células dendríticas activadas, macrófagos y células epiteliales, tiene efectos complejos sobre el sistema inmunitario. Sus acciones inflamatorias son:

- Promueve la diferenciación de nuestros linfocitos CD4 TH1 mediante la inducción del factor de transcripción T-bet, para así combatir microbios intracelulares y células tumorales malignas.

- Favorece la activación de nuestros linfocitos NK.

Luna también tiene efectos antiinflamatorios:

- Inhibe la inmunidad TH17 actuando a través de STAT1.

- Induce la síntesis de IL-10 para activar linfocitos T reguladores.

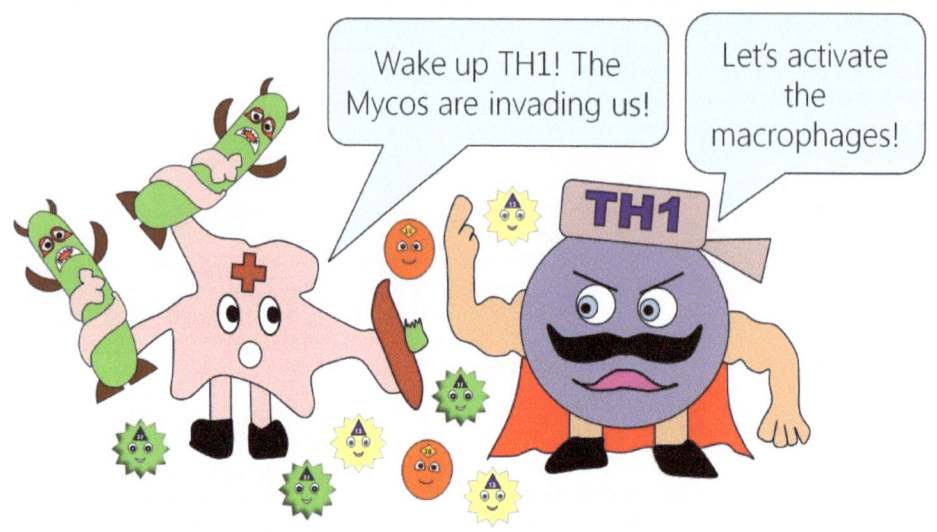

Are there people who cannot produce IL-27?

Patients with absent or reduced STAT1 function have impaired signaling of several TH1 cytokines (e.g. interferon-γ, IL-27, interferons α and β), becoming susceptible to infections by intracellular microorganisms such as mycobacteria and viruses.

Are there people who fabricate IL-27 in excess?

Patients with STAT1 gain-of-function mutations are characterized by an excessive activity of interferons and IL-27, which results in:

- Susceptibility to infections by extracellular fungi and bacteria, as a consequence of a weak TH17 army.

- Autoimmune phenomena such as lupus-like syndrome.

Lili and Lali, the interleukins 28

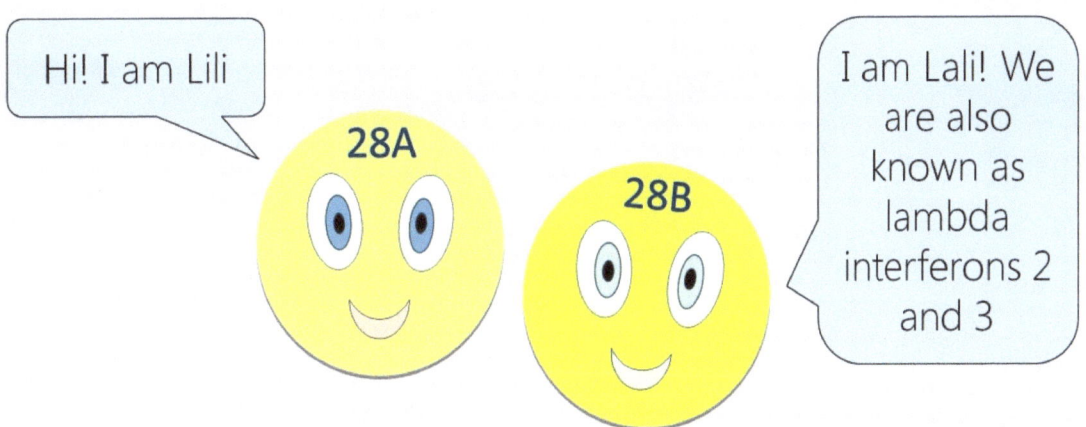

Lili is our interleukin 28A, also known as interferon-lambda 2 (IFN-λ2). Her sister Lali is our IL-28B (IFN-λ3). Both belong to the IL-10 family, together with interleukins 10, 19, 20, 22, 24, 26 and 29.

Both sisters exert their actions, essentially antiviral, through a receptor formed by the chains IL-28R1 and IL-10R2.

Where are they produced?

Lili and Lali are synthesized by various cells, mainly dendritic cells, in response to viral attacks, in order to enhance our TH1 immune army. Both cytokines are capable of inhibiting the replication of hepatitis B and C viruses, as well as stimulating the destruction of cancer cells.

On the other hand, Lili and Lali may contribute to the development of tolerogenic dendritic cells, capable of inducing T regulatory lymphocytes.

Both cytokines have inhibitory activity over the TH2 immune army.

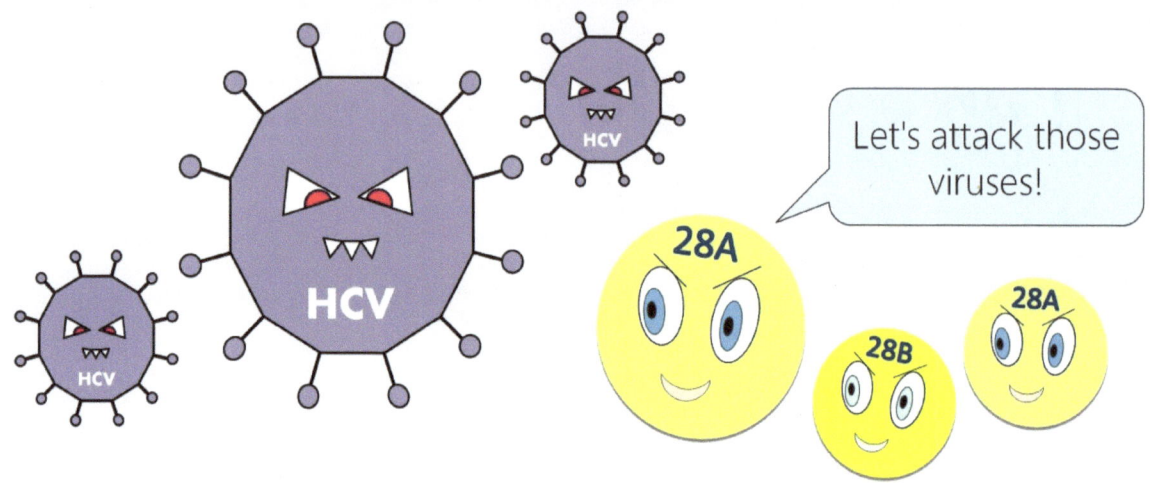

Are there people who cannot produce IL-28?

Genetic immunodeficiencies caused by absence of IL-28 have not been described.

Certain polymorphisms in the IL-28B gene predict clinical response to hepatitis C treatment with ribavirin plus interferon α.

After reviewing their actions, we deduce that Lili and Lali have therapeutic potential against viral infections, malignant tumors and allergic diseases.

Are there people who fabricate IL-28 in excess?

Unnecessary production of IL-28A or IL-28B may favor the development of autoimmune diseases such as Sjögren's syndrome.

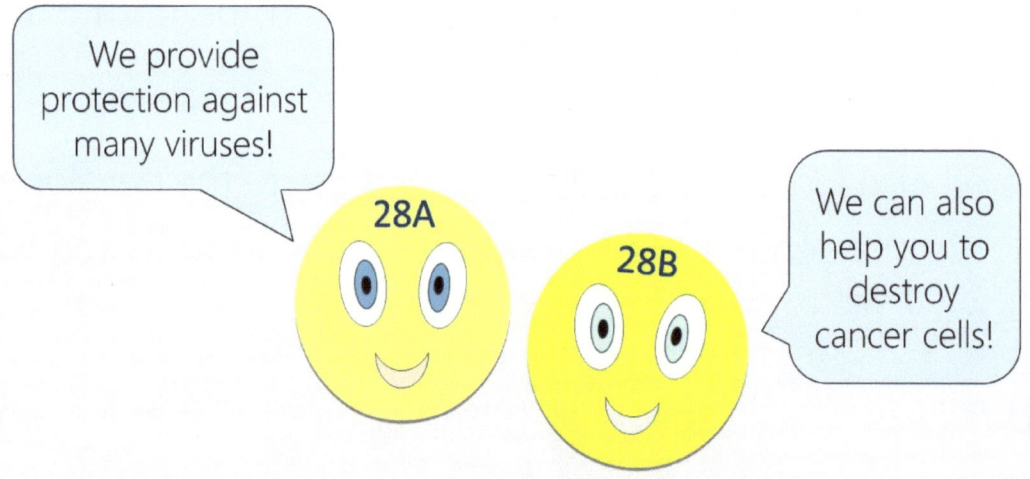

Areli, the interleukin 29

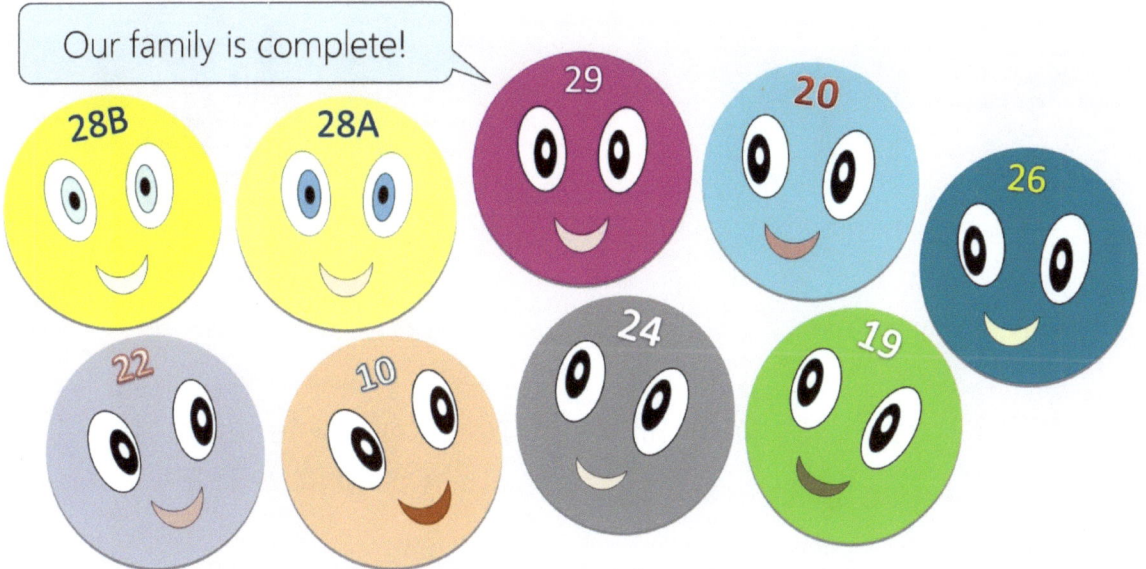

Areli, our beautiful interleukin-29, also called IFN-λ1, completes the family of interferons type III (lambda interferons) together with Lili and Lali (interleukins 28A and 28B). All of them fulfill their functions through a receptor formed by the chains IL-28R1 and IL-10R2.

Areli is also part of the IL-10 family, together with interleukins 10, 19, 20, 22, 24, 26 and 28.

Where is Areli produced?

Areli is produced by several cells, mainly dendritic cells, in response to viral attack, aiming to boost our TH1 defense army. Like her sisters Lili and Lali, Areli has antiviral and antitumor effects.

Other important actions of Areli are: contribution to the development of tolerogenic dendritic cells, and inhibition of the TH2 immune army.

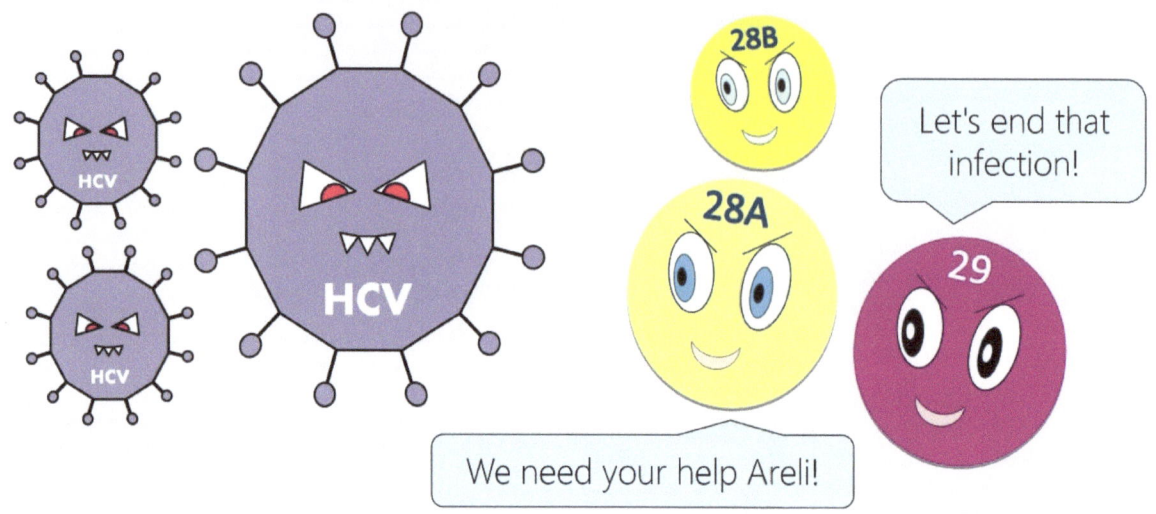

Are there people who cannot produce IL-29?

To date, no patients with clinically relevant defects in the IL-29 gene have been reported.

Pegylated Interferon Lambda-1a has inhibitory activity against hepatitis C virus. Other potential applications of this drug are cancer and severe allergies.

Are there people who fabricate IL-29 in excess?

Local excess of IL-29 synthesis may favor the development of autoimmune diseases such as systemic lupus erythematosus, multiple sclerosis, and rheumatoid arthritis.

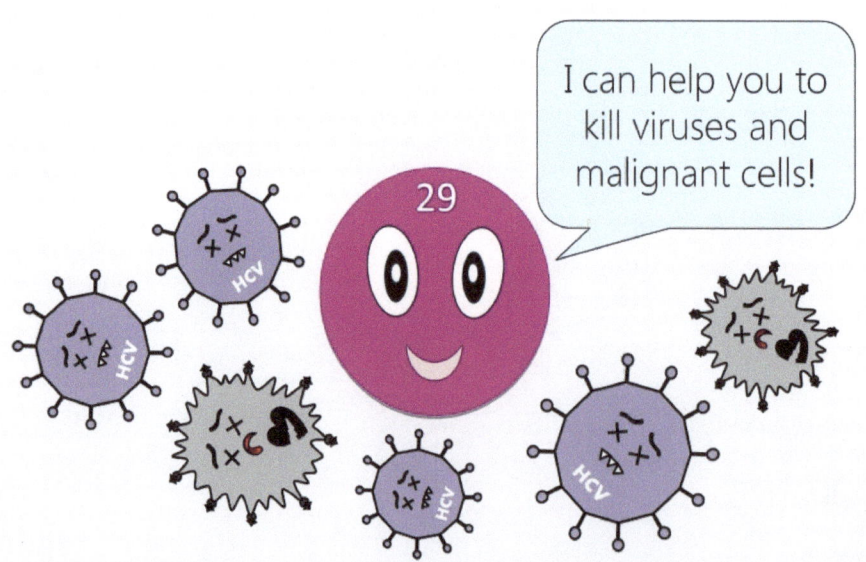

Fanny, the interleukin 30

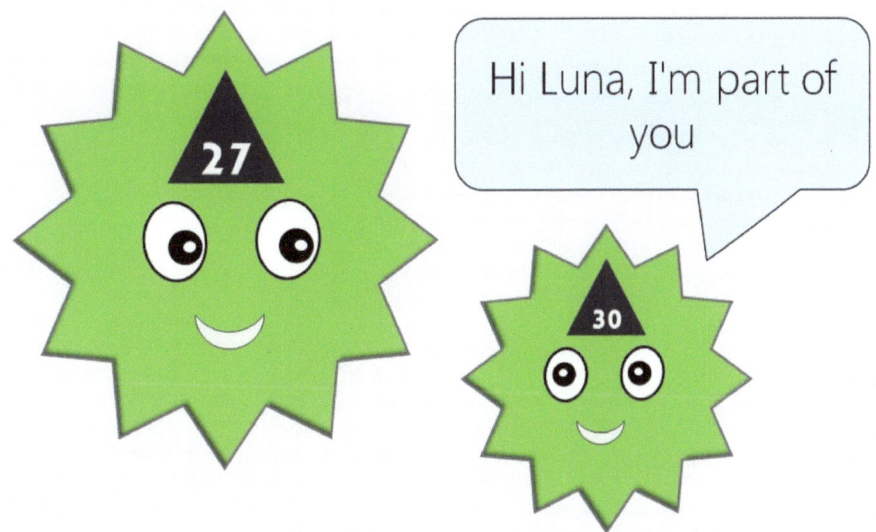

Fanny, our interleukin 30, is the p28 subunit of Luna, our interleukin 27.

Where is Fanny produced?

IL-30 is a potent anti-inflammatory cytokine. Its best known role is the prevention and treatment of liver damage caused by inflammatory phenomena.

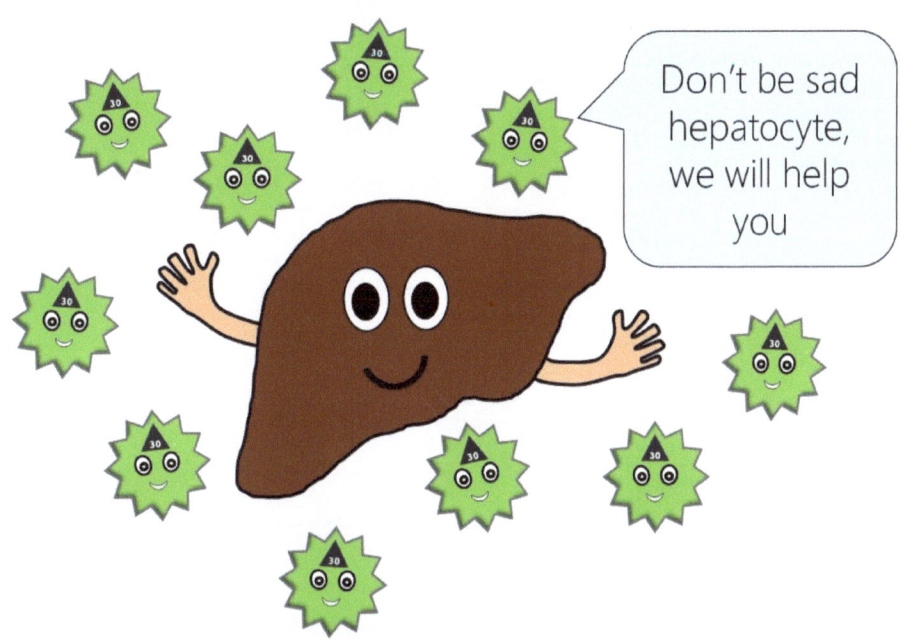

Are there people who cannot produce IL-30?

Primary immunodeficiencies due to lack of interleukin 30 have not been described.

The anti-inflammatory effect of IL-30 can be harnessed for the management of patients with sepsis.

Are there people who fabricate IL-30 in excess?

Local overload of interleukin 30 could inhibit the attack of our immune system to malignant cells, becoming a risk factor for the appearance of cancer.

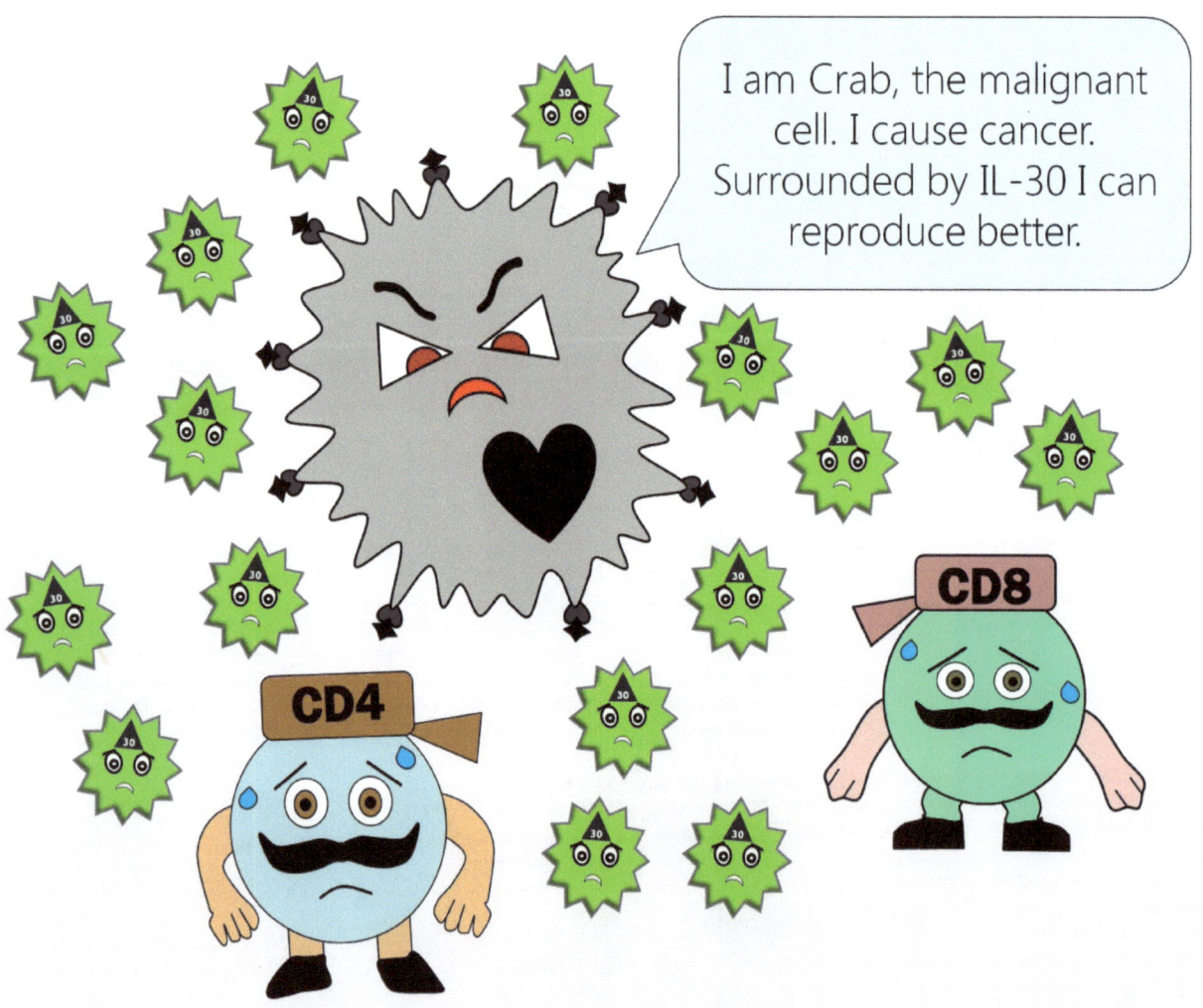

Rachel, the interleukin 31

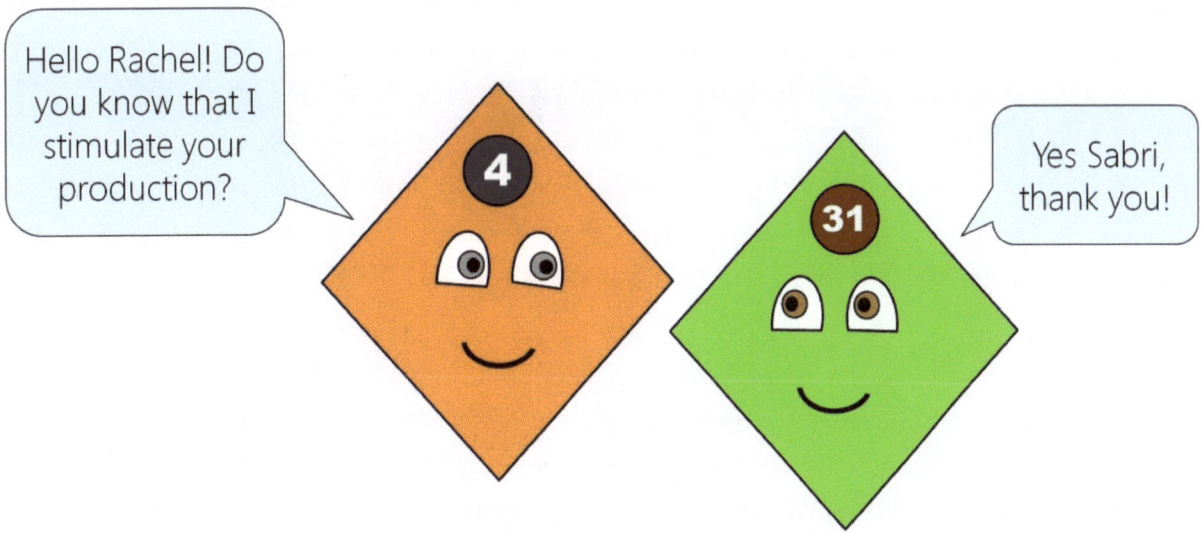

Our interleukin 31 is a TH2 inflammatory cytokine whose most prominent role is generation of pruritus. Its receptor is made up of two subunits: IL-31RA and OSMRβ (oncostatin M receptor β).

Where is Rachel produced?

Rachel is synthesized by activated T lymphocytes, both CD4 and CD8, especially by TH2 commanders. Her production is stimulated by the action of IL-4. Other cells capable of making IL-31 are monocytes, macrophages, dendritic cells, mast cells, keratinocytes and fibroblasts.

Rachel has several actions that increase TH2 inflammation:

- Activates the sensation of pruritus by acting on receptors in the peripheral sensory nerve cells.

- Induces the production of inflammatory chemokines by eosinophils and epithelial cells including keratinocytes.

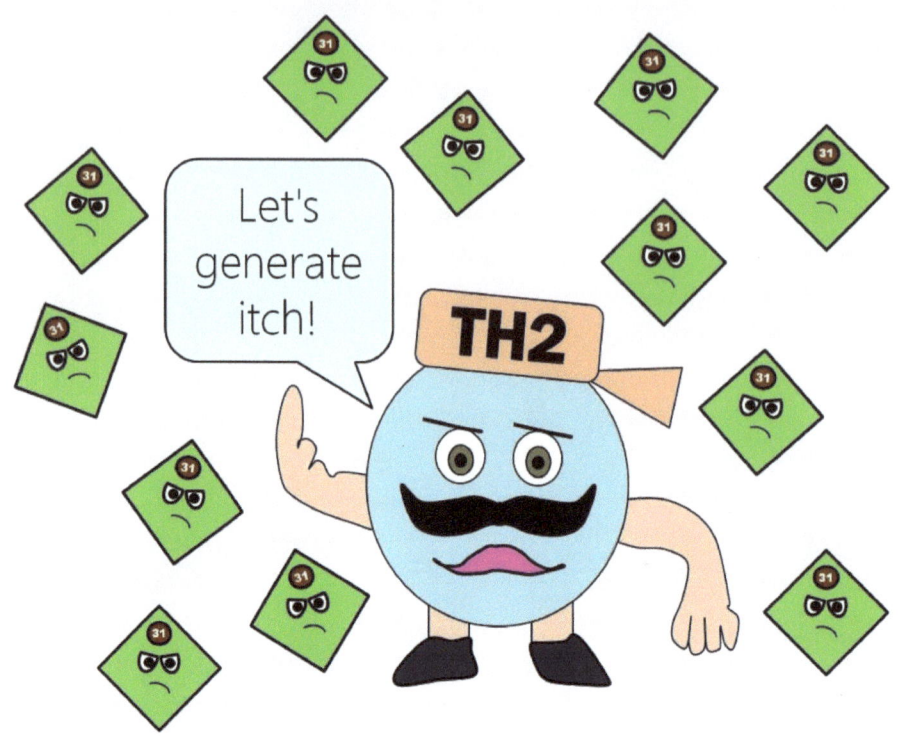

Are there people who cannot produce IL-31?

Immunodeficiencies due to IL-31 absence have not been reported.

Are there people who fabricate IL-31 in excess?

IL-31 favors the development and progression of inflammatory diseases with pruritus (e.g. atopic and non-atopic dermatitis, contact dermatitis, prurigo, chronic urticaria, mastocytosis).

In patients affected by these pathologies, IL-31 is a potential marker of severity, as well as a therapeutic target.

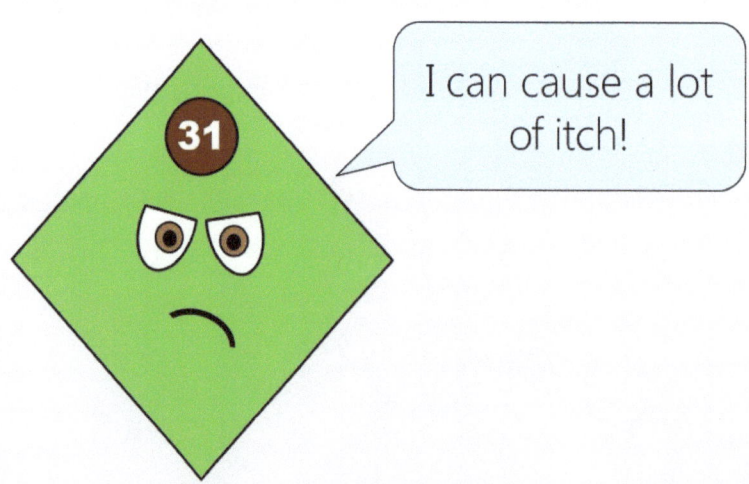

Gabi, the interleukin 32

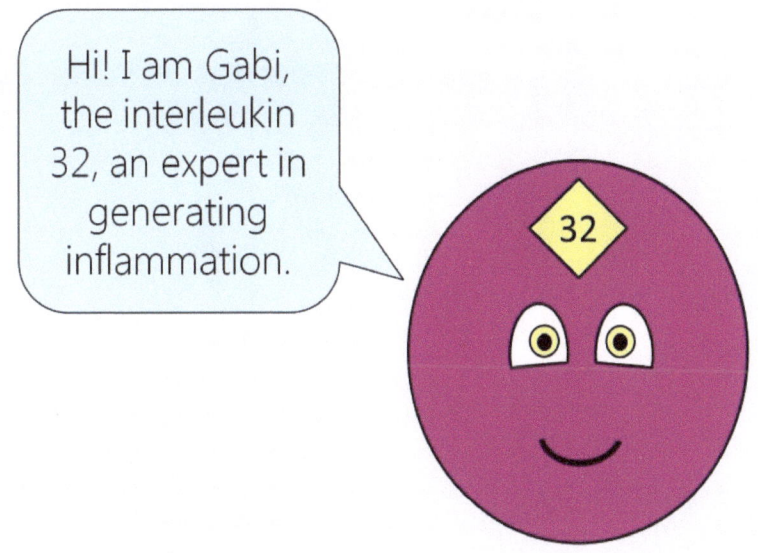

Now we will meet Gabi, our powerful interleukin 32. Its action is essentially proinflammatory. To date, its receptors have not been defined.

Where is Gabi produced?

Several cells are able to synthesize IL-32, including monocytes, macrophages, NK lymphocytes, T lymphocytes and epithelial cells.

Gabi induces the production of other inflammatory cytokines such as interleukin 6, interleukin 8 and tumor necrosis factor-α (TNF-α). It also promotes apoptosis of epithelial cells and osteoclast differentiation.

Are there people who cannot produce IL-32?

Immunodeficiencies because of IL-32 absence have not been described yet.

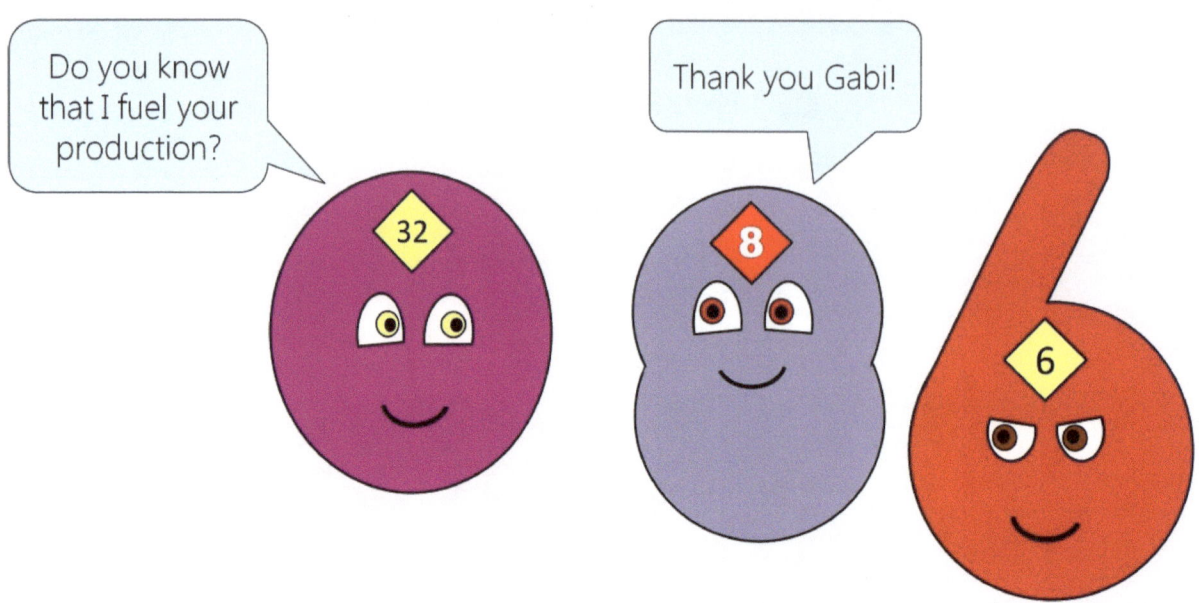

Are there people who fabricate IL-32 in excess?

Excessive activity of interleukin 32 in healthy tissues may lead to the development of chronic inflammatory diseases such as rheumatoid arthritis, inflammatory bowel disease, chronic rhinosinusitis, atopic dermatitis and cancer.

In these diseases, IL-32 can serve as a biomarker of severity and as a therapeutic target.

To date, anti-IL-32 monoclonal antibodies have not been developed.

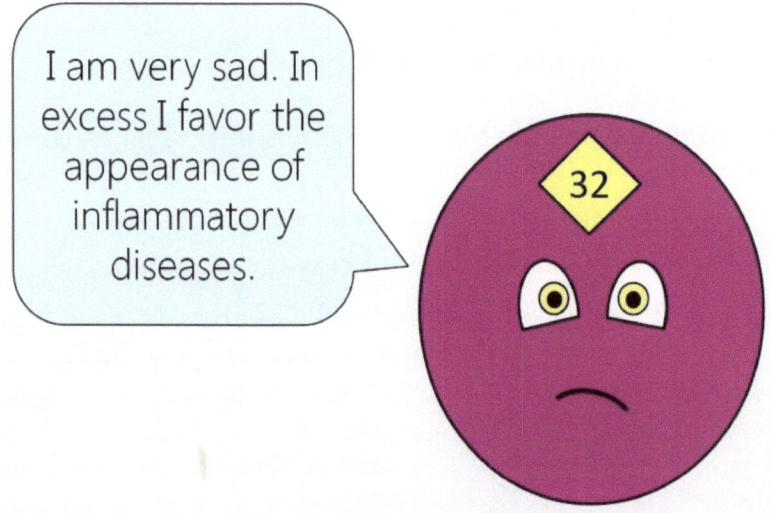

Techi, the interleukin 33

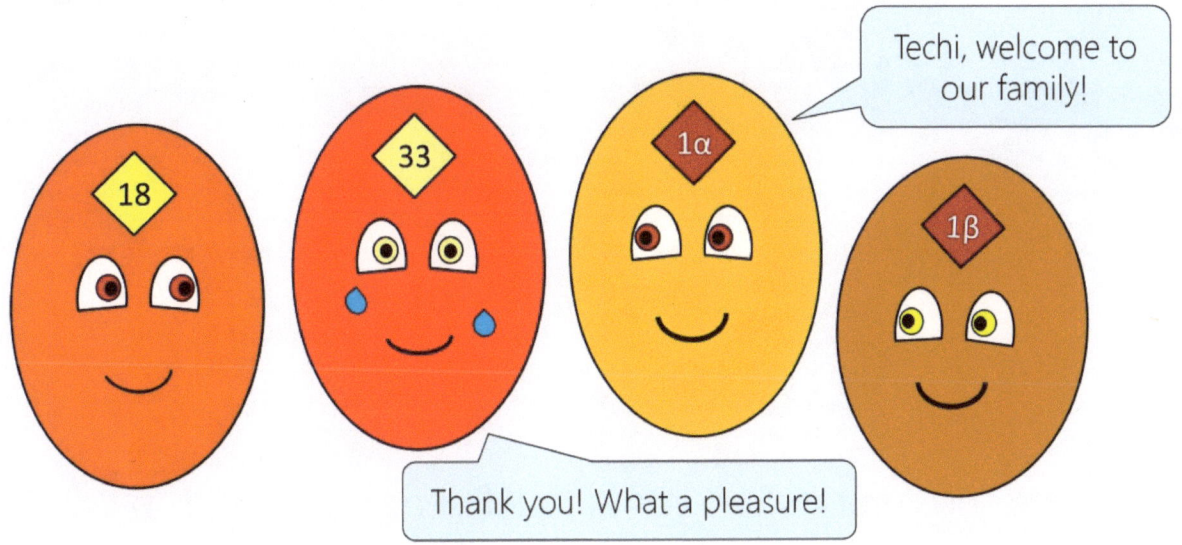

IL-33 is a member of IL-1 family, along with other six inflammatory cytokines (IL-1α, IL-1β, IL-18, IL-36α, IL-36β, IL-36γ) and four anti-inflammatory interleukins (IL-1Ra, IL-36Ra, IL-37, IL-38).

Techi stimulates TH2 immunity through the receptor ST2, which also has regulatory function in its soluble form.

Where is Techi produced?

Techi is produced by epithelial cells (e.g. keratinocytes) and stromal cells (e.g. fibroblasts) in response to cell damage. She is also released from necrotic cells to promote inflammation, thus fulfilling her role of 'alarmin'.

Techi has multiple inflammatory actions. She induces maturation of proinflammatory dendritic cells, stimulates type 2 innate lymphoid cells, and promotes activation of basophils, eosinophils and mast cells.

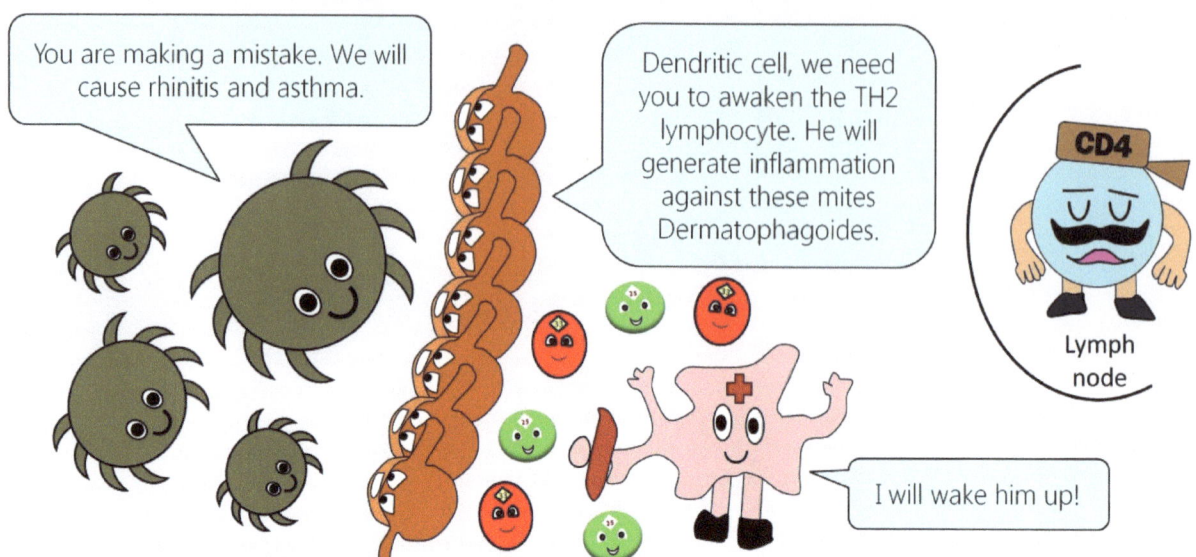

Are there people who cannot produce IL-33?

There are no reports of immunodeficiencies caused by IL-33 absence.

Are there people who fabricate IL-33 in excess?

Excessive production of IL-33, conditioned by genetic variants and environmental factors (e.g. viruses, cigarette smoke, environmental pollutants), favors the development of inflammatory diseases such as bronchial asthma and atopic dermatitis.

Certain viral infections activate bronchial epithelial cells to produce the TH2-inducing cytokines IL-33, IL-25 and TSLP (thymic stromal lymphopoietin).

IL-33 can damage the skin barrier by reducing filaggrin expression.

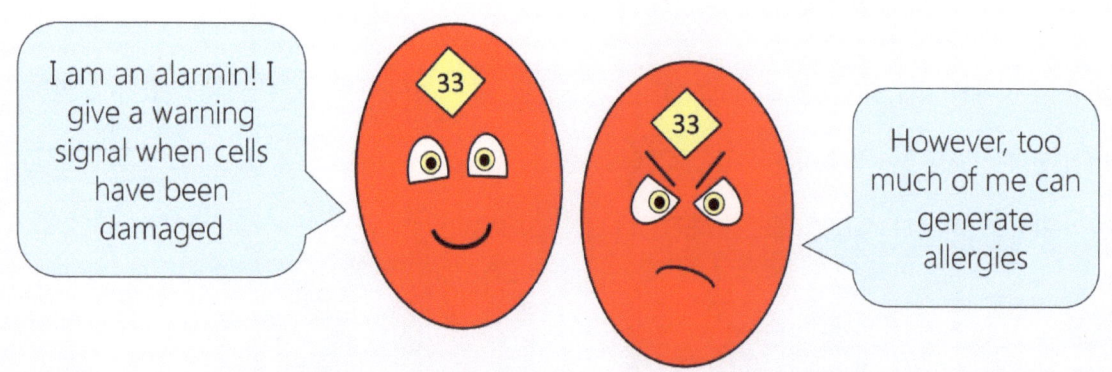

Gina, the interleukin 34

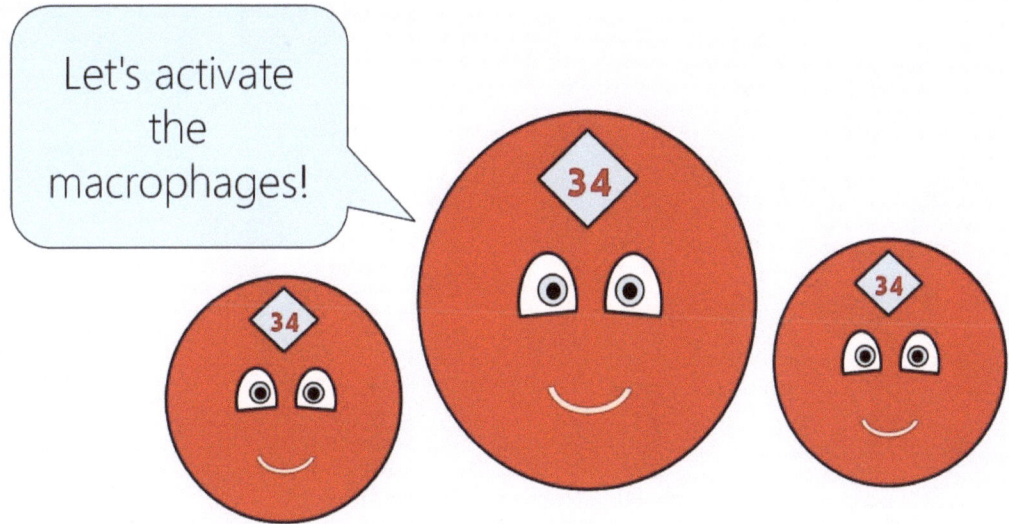

We will now study Gina, our interleukin 34. This proinflammatory cytokine acts through the receptor named CSF1R ('colony-stimulating factor 1 receptor'). CSF1R also mediates CSF1 signaling.

Where is Gina produced?

Gina is manufactured in the spleen, liver, heart, brain, kidneys, thymus, ovaries, testes, prostate, skin and intestines.

She induces the differentiation, proliferation and survival of monocytes/macrophages, microglia, osteoclasts and Langerhans cells, thereby promoting inflammatory response.

Are there people who cannot produce IL-34?

Patients with primary immunodeficiencies caused by lack of IL-34 have not been reported yet.

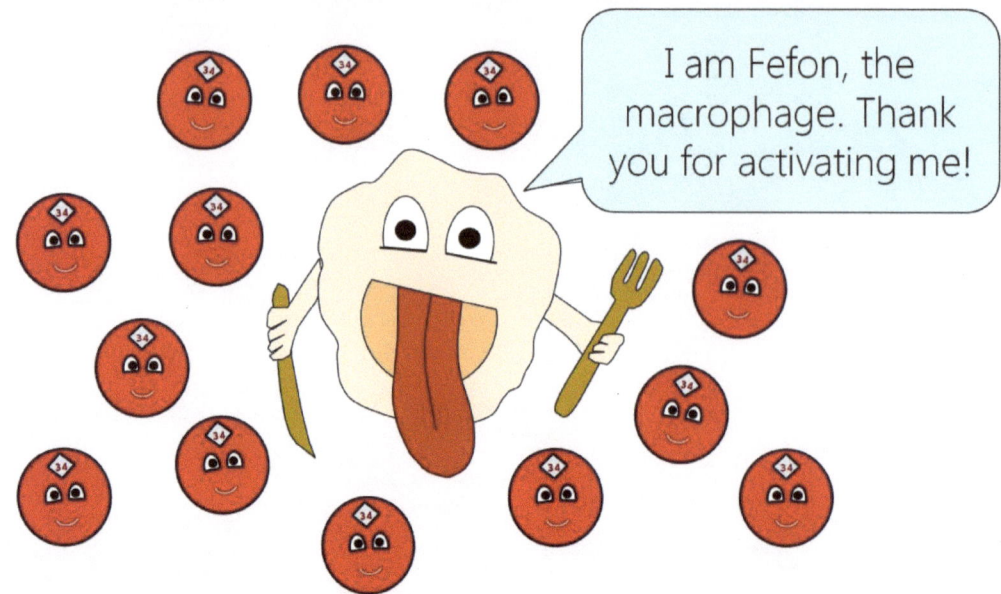

Are there people who fabricate IL-34 in excess?

IL-34 overload may favor the development of inflammatory diseases (e.g. rheumatoid arthritis, inflammatory bowel disease, pigmented vellonodular synovitis).

Cabiralizumab is an anti-CSF1R monoclonal antibody that blocks the action of IL-34 and CSF1. It has therapeutic potential for patients affected by monocyte-induced inflammatory diseases.

In addition, the combination of Cabiralizumab and Nivolumab (anti-PD-1 monoclonal antibody) is being evaluated for the treatment of neoplasms. The basis of this therapy is to inhibit the development of pro-tumor macrophages.

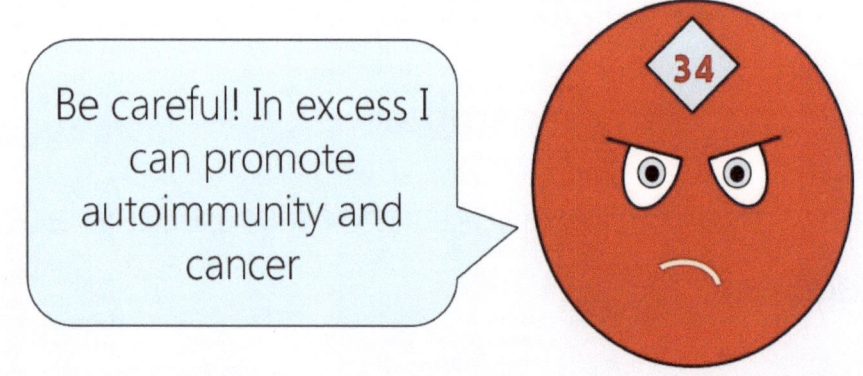

Carla, the interleukin 35

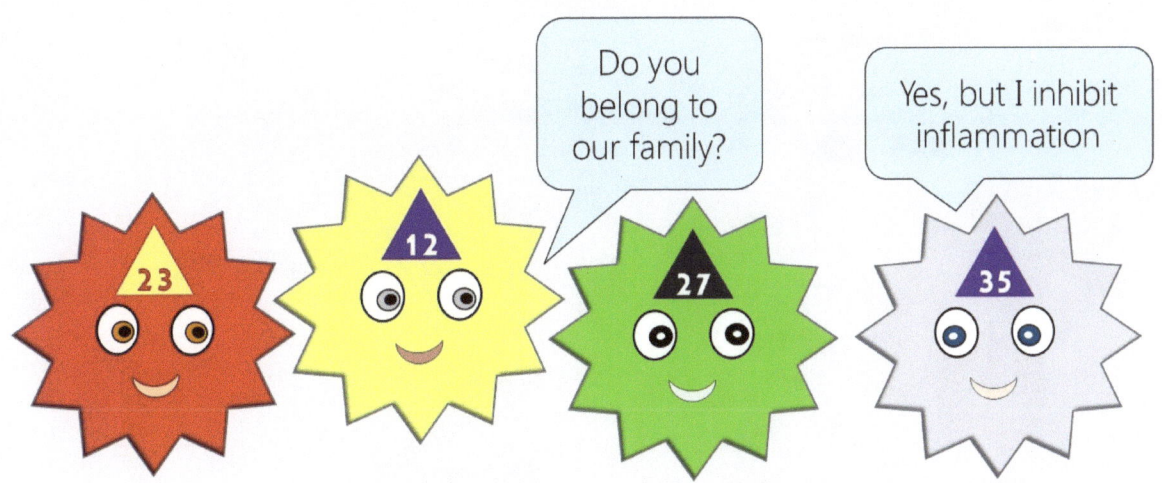

Carla is a member of the IL-12 family, along with interleukins 12, 23 and 27. However, unlike her sisters, Carla has anti-inflammatory actions.

Carla has 2 subunits: p35 (it is also part of Bolli, our interleukin 12) and EBI3 (it also makes up Luna, our interleukin 27).

IL-35 receptors are formed by the combination of the IL-12Rβ2 and gp130 chains (IL-12Rβ2/gp130, IL-12Rβ2/IL-12Rβ2 and gp130/gp130). Remind that IL-12Rβ2 is also part of the IL-12 receptor and that gp130 also builds the receptors of interleukins 6, 11 and 27.

Where is Carla produced?

Carla is synthesized by T regulatory lymphocytes, monocytes, endothelial and epithelial cells. Her major actions are:

- Inhibition of inflammatory effector T lymphocytes.
- Activation of T and B regulatory lymphocytes.

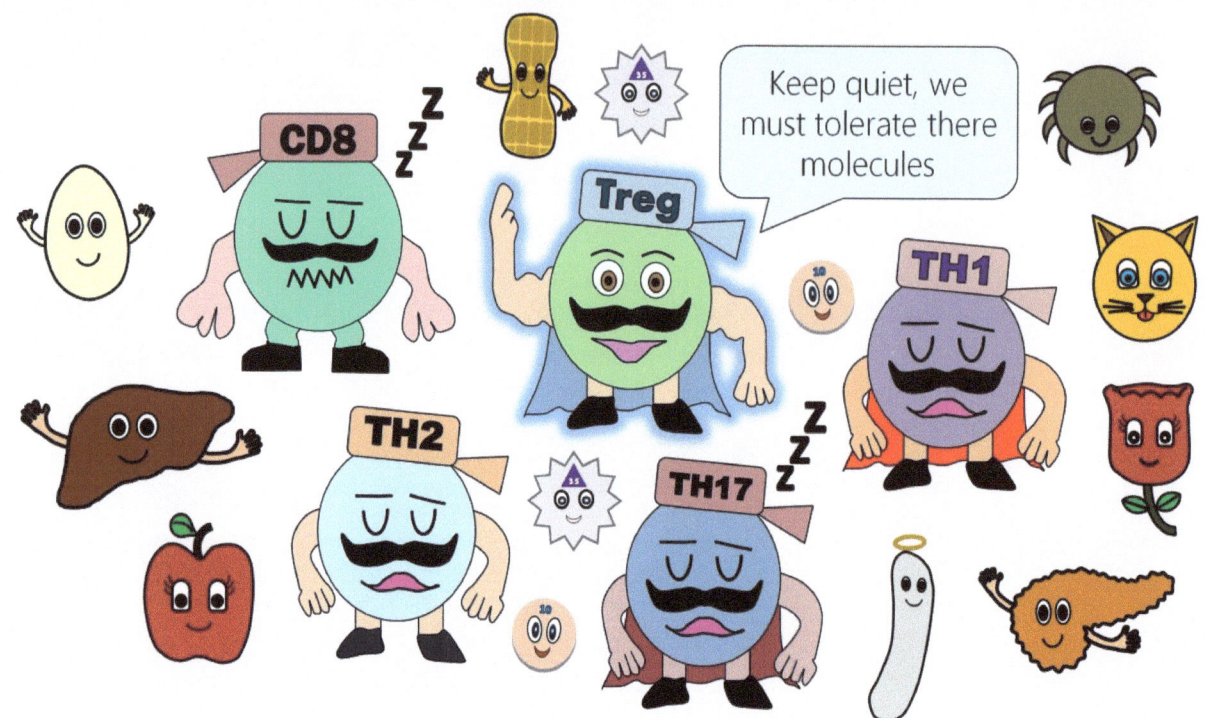

Are there people who cannot produce IL-35?

Children lacking T regulatory lymphocytes have early-onset autoimmunity. For example, patients with Foxp3 deficiency develop IPEX syndrome (immune dysregulation, autoimmune polyendocrinopathy, enteropathy, X-linked).

Local deficit of IL-35 can facilitate the development of autoimmune and allergic diseases. Recombinant IL-35 could play a therapeutic role in these diseases.

Are there people who fabricate IL-35 in excess?

Local excess of IL-35 may favor the progression of cancer.

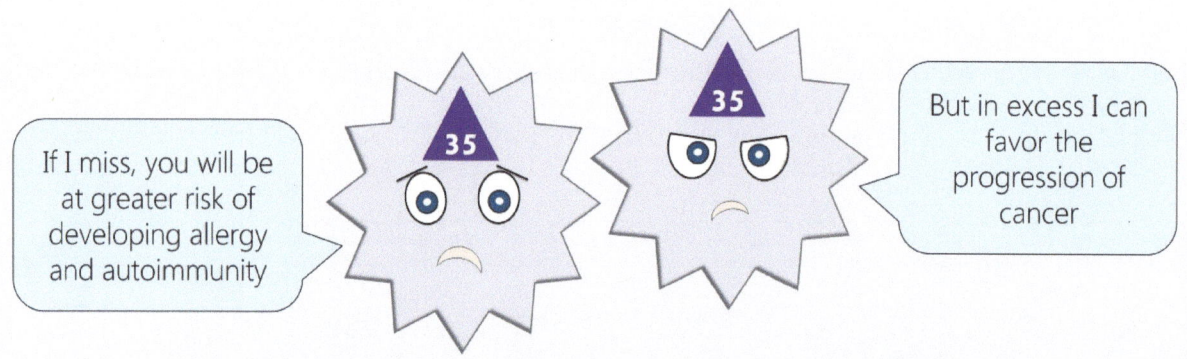

Adela, IL-36α, and her family

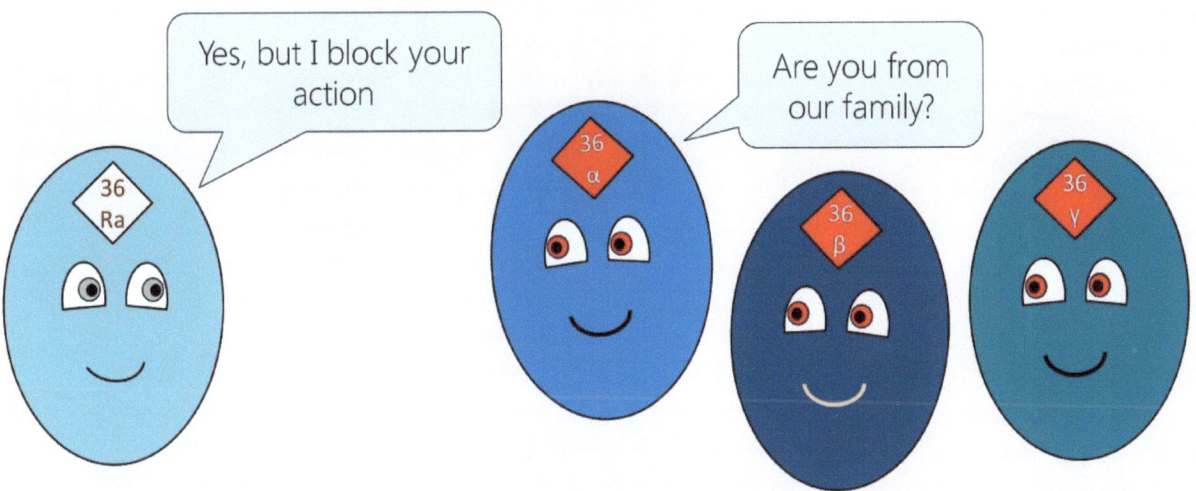

There are four subtypes of interleukin 36: three have inflammatory activity (IL-36α, IL-36β, IL-36γ) and one is the natural antagonist (IL-36Ra or IL-36 receptor antagonist). All of them belong to the interleukin-1 family.

IL-36 receptor consists of 2 subunits: IL-36R and IL-1RAP (Interleukin-1 receptor accessory protein).

Where are they produced?

Adela and her sisters are synthesized by epithelial and endothelial cells, especially in the skin, as well as by macrophages.

Our cytokines IL-36α, IL-36β and IL-36γ are proinflammatory; they induce innate immune response following tissue damage. In addition, they favor proliferation of T lymphocytes and differentiation towards TH1/TH17 lymphocytes.

In contrast, IL-36Ra has anti-inflammatory activity by antagonizing the action of IL-36α, IL-36β and IL-36γ.

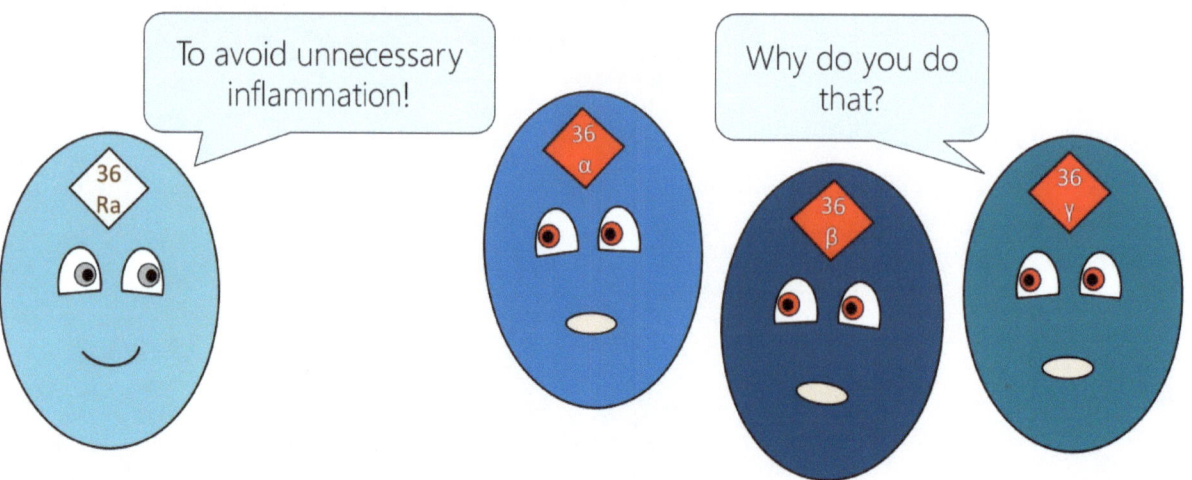

Are there people who cannot produce IL-36?

There are people who cannot make IL-36Ra. The resulting disease is called DITRA (Deficiency of the Interleukin 36 Receptor Antagonist), characterized by early-onset generalized pustular psoriasis (fever, pustular rash, leukocytosis, elevation of acute phase reactants).

Are there people who fabricate IL-36 in excess?

Excessive synthesis of IL-36α, IL-36β or IL-36γ favors the development of severe forms of psoriasis.

Affected patients may benefit from biological therapies that neutralize these cytokines or their receptor (e.g. ANB019, an anti-IL-36R monoclonal antibody, still under investigation).

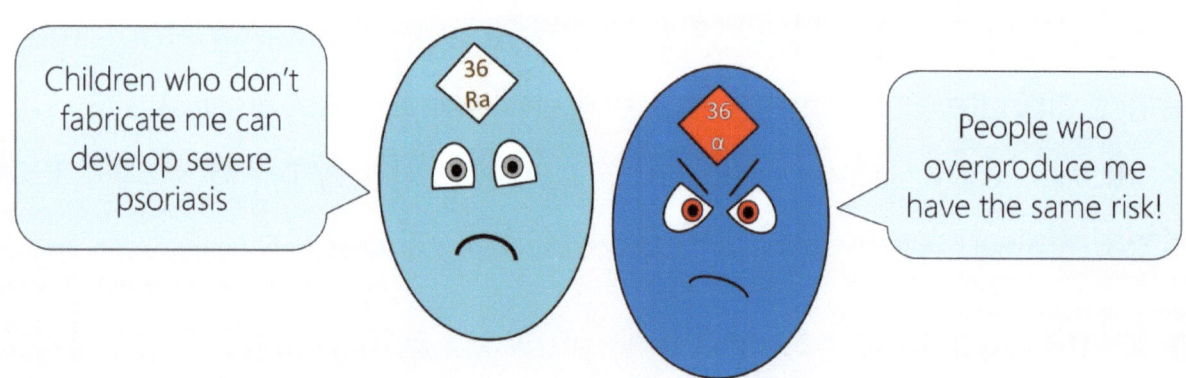

Ethel, the interleukin 37

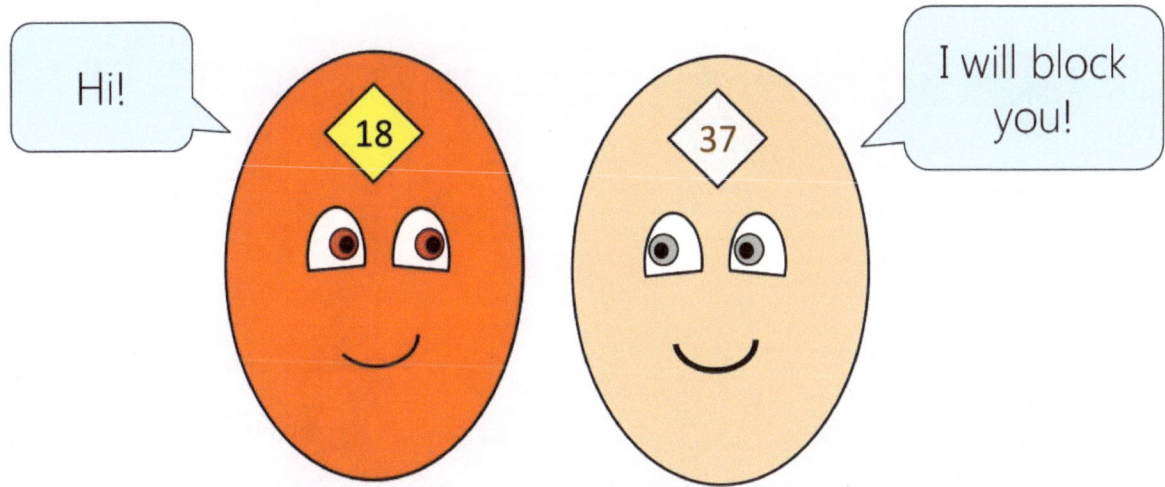

IL-37 is an anti-inflammatory cytokine that antagonizes IL-18. Remind that both molecules belong to the interleukin-1 family, together with other pro-inflammatory (IL-1α, IL-1β, IL-33, IL-36α, IL-36β, IL-36γ) and anti-inflammatory cytokines (IL-1Ra, IL-36Ra, IL-38).

Ethel exerts her functions through the molecules IL-18Rα and the inhibitory component IL-1R8 (IL-1 receptor family member 8).

Where is Ethel produced?

Interleukin 37 is synthesized by monocytes. In addition, various tumor cells are capable of producing this cytokine, perhaps to escape from the attack of the immune system.

Ethel has anti-inflammatory actions, which include:

- Antagonism of IL-18.
- Inhibition of dendritic cells.

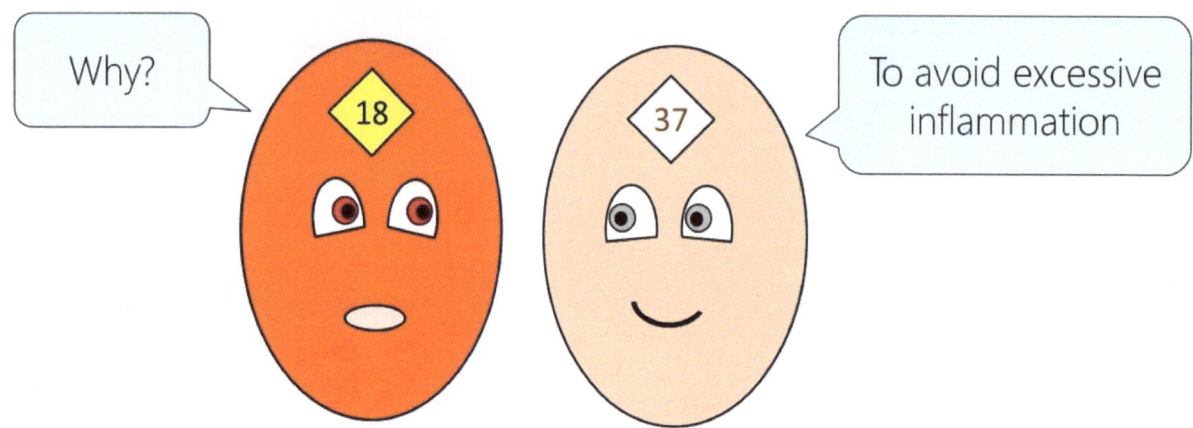

Are there people who cannot produce IL-37?

Local decrease of IL-37 could favor the onset or progression of inflammatory diseases such as rheumatoid arthritis, ankylosing spondylitis and systemic lupus erythematosus.

Patients affected by these diseases could benefit from the use of recombinant human IL-37.

Are there people who fabricate IL-37 in excess?

Local excess of IL-37 may be a risk factor for the development of infections (e.g. tuberculosis) or cancer (e.g. squamous cell carcinoma). A pro-angiogenic role of IL-37 in proliferative retinopathy has been described.

However, it has also been reported that IL-37 might have antitumor effect by inhibiting angiogenesis.

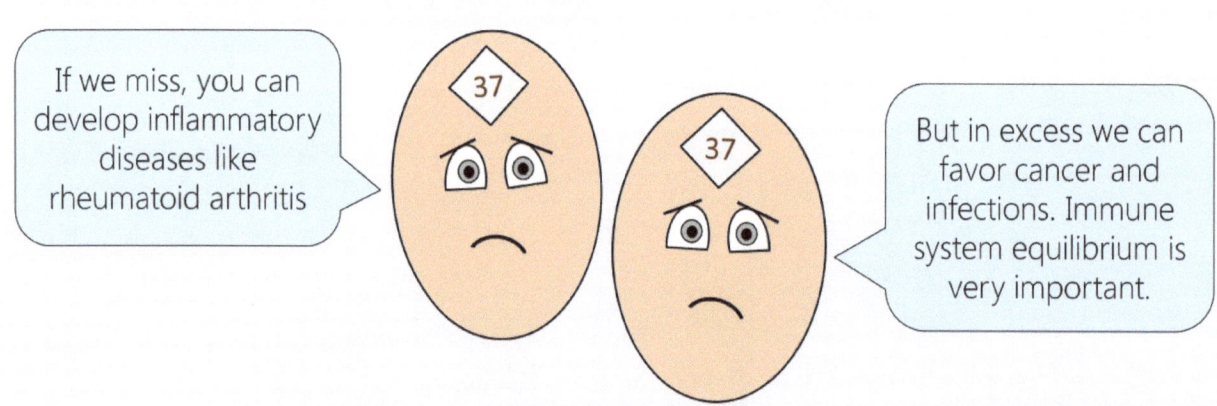

Gladys, the interleukin 38

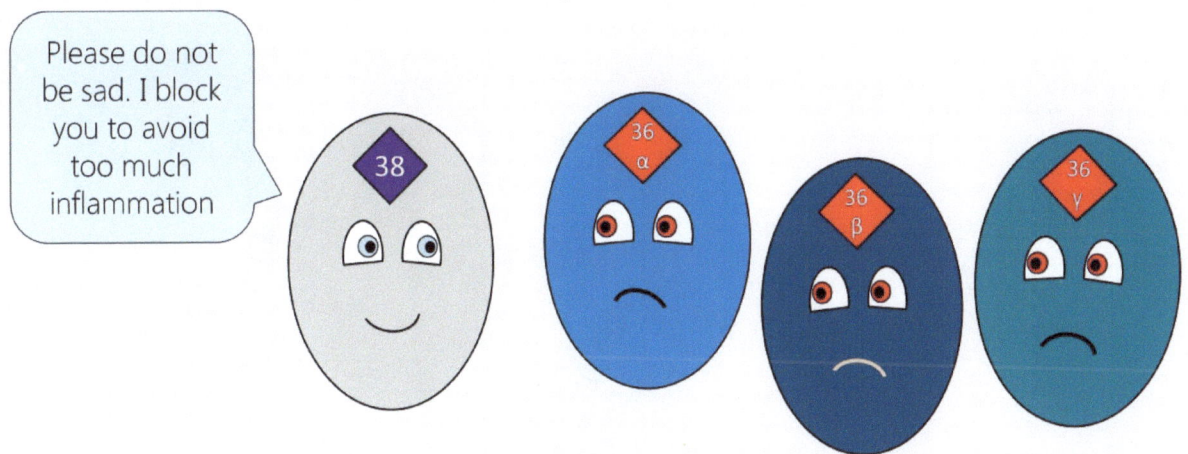

Let's welcome Gladys, our interleukin 38! Like her sister Ethel, Gladys is an anti-inflammatory cytokine. Interleukin-38 is the last of the 11 members of the interleukin-1 family (IL-1α, IL-1β, IL-1Ra, IL-18, IL-33, IL-36α, IL-36β, IL-36γ, IL-36Rα, IL-37 and IL-38).

IL-38 exerts her actions through IL-36R and, to a lesser extent, through IL-1R1 (interleukin-1 receptor type 1).

Where is Gladys produced?

Gladys can be synthesized in several tissues such as the skin, spleen, placenta, thymus, tonsils and salivary glands.

Gladys, whose structure is similar to the molecules IL-1Ra and IL-36Ra, has the following anti-inflammatory actions:

- Antagonizes the inflammatory action of IL-36.

- Inhibits the activation of TH17 immunity, including the production of IL-17, IL-22 and IL-8.

- Es liberada por células apoptóticas para limitar la respuesta inflamatoria de los macrófagos.

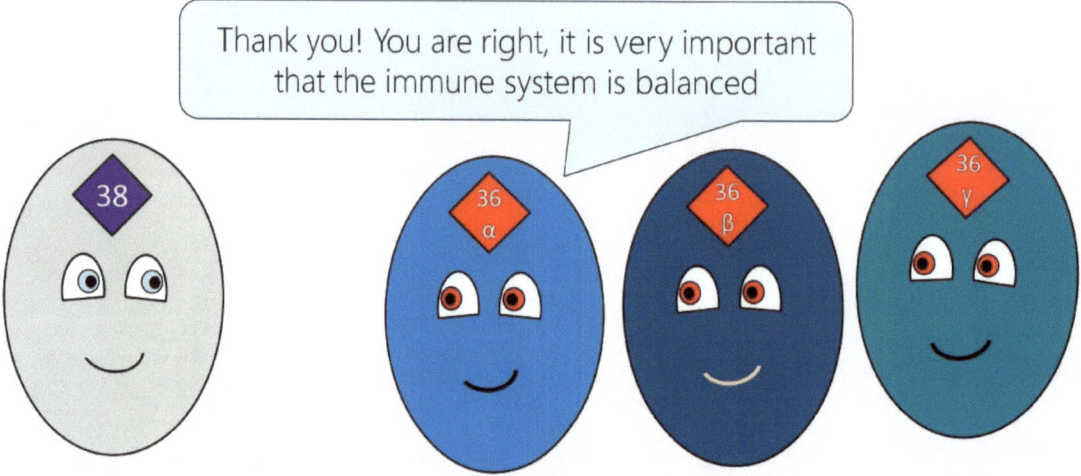

Are there people who cannot produce IL-38?

Genetic polymorphisms that reduce the synthesis or activity of IL-38 may favor the development of inflammatory diseases (e.g. rheumatoid arthritis, systemic lupus erythematosus).

Recombinant IL-38 has a potential therapeutic role in these diseases.

Are there people who fabricate IL-38 in excess?

Given its immunosuppressive effect, local excess of IL-38 could favor the development of infections and cancer.

Elevated levels of IL-38 have been reported to predict a better response to telbivudine in patients with chronic hepatitis B.

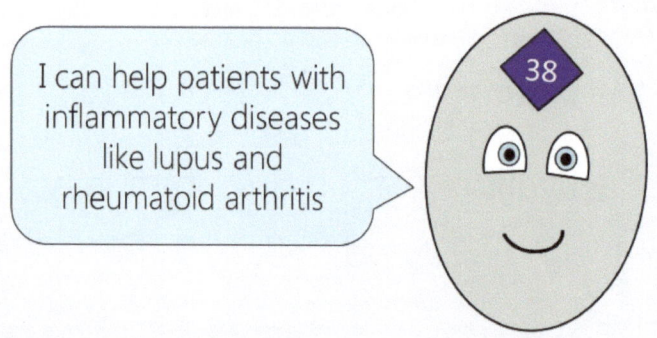

In this book we have learned about the role of interleukins in the normal function of our immune system and in distinct immunological diseases (immunodeficiencies, autoimmunity, allergies, autoinflammation and cancer).

Do not miss our next educational books, where we will continue learning on the fantastic world of Immunology.

Juan Carlos Aldave, MD
Allergy and Clinical Immunology

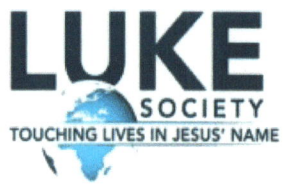 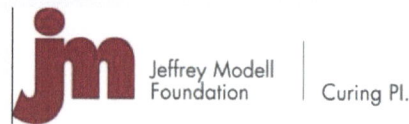

Contributors:

- Juan Félix Aldave Pita, MD
- Bertha Alicia Becerra Sánchez
- Ana Ponce de León Camahualí

Sponsors:

- Jeffrey Modell Foundation
- Luke Society International

"For God so loved the world that he gave his one and only Son, that whoever believes in him shall not perish but have eternal life". John 3:16

10 Warning Signs of Primary Immunodeficiency

Primary Immunodeficiency (PI) causes children and adults to have infections that come back frequently or are unusually hard to cure. 1:500 persons are affected by one of the known Primary Immunodeficiencies. **If you or someone you know is affected by two or more of the following Warning Signs, speak to a physician about the possible presence of an underlying Primary Immunodeficiency.**

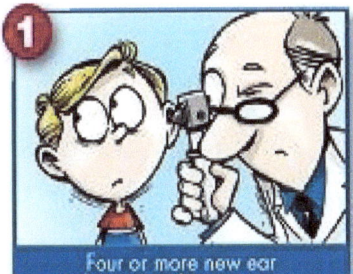
1. Four or more new ear infections within one year.

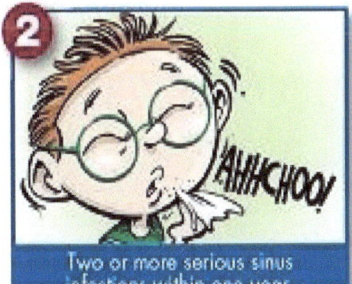
2. Two or more serious sinus infections within one year.

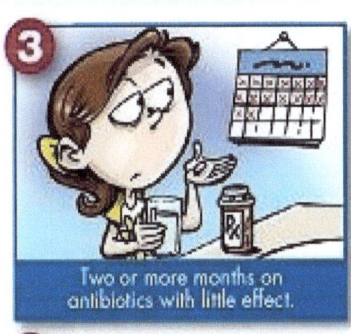
3. Two or more months on antibiotics with little effect.

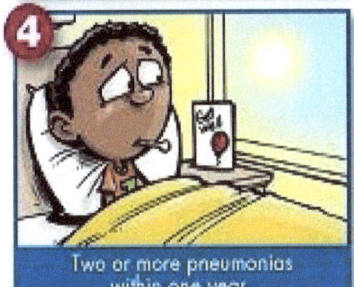
4. Two or more pneumonias within one year.

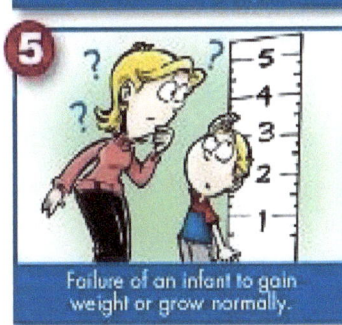
5. Failure of an infant to gain weight or grow normally.

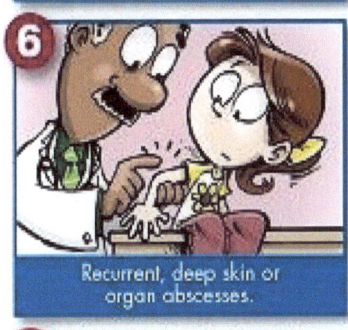
6. Recurrent, deep skin or organ abscesses.

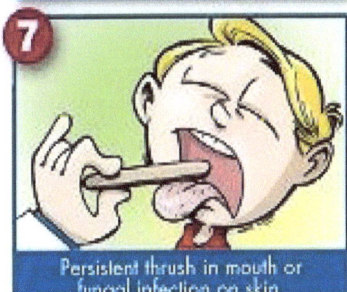
7. Persistent thrush in mouth or fungal infection on skin.

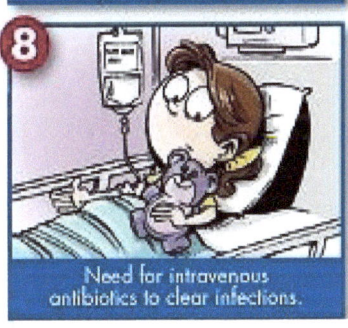
8. Need for intravenous antibiotics to clear infections.

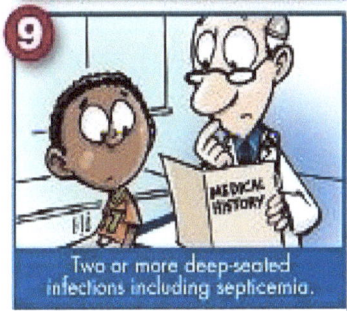
9. Two or more deep-seated infections including septicemia.

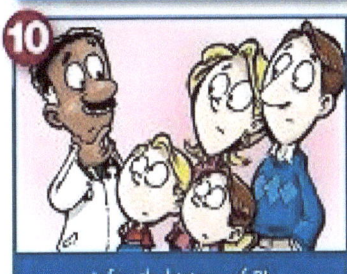
10. A family history of PI.

"These warning signs were developed by the Jeffrey Modell Foundation Medical Advisory Board. Consultation with Primary Immunodeficiency experts is strongly suggested.
©2013 Jeffrey Modell Foundation"

www.INFO4PI.org

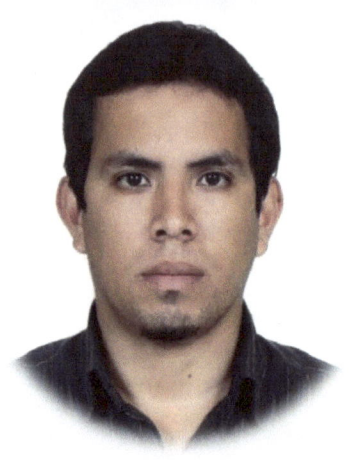

Juan Carlos Aldave, MD
Allergy and Clinical Immunology

"Proper functioning of our immune system is essential for life. The purpose of this book series is to introduce everyone into the fantastic world of Immunology".

Book series: Funny Immunology to Save Lives
(Editions in English and Spanish)

- Book 1: The Immunocytes
- Book 2: The TH17 army against Candida
- Book 3: The TH1 army against Mycobacteria
- Book 4: The TH2 army against worms
- Book 5: The battle against Pneumococcus
- Book 6: The Immunocytes against cancer
- Book 7: T regs: controlling the immune army
- Book 8: When the Immunocytes get sick...
- Book 9: When the Immunocytes go crazy...
- Book 10: The Immunocytes and transplantation
- Book 11: The armor of the Immunocyte Felix
- Book 12: The fantastic Interleukins

Contact the Author:
Jirón Domingo Cueto 371, Of. 301, Lince, LIMA 14
Lima, Perú
Phones: +51 948-323-720
+51 988-689-472
jucapul_84@hotmail.com
funny.immunology@gmail.com
www.alergomed.org/immunocytes